# The Winner's Manual

*Take Control of Your Life*

**Bobby Lynch**

How to Ditch the Quick Fixes and Finally
Produce Results That Last!

IngramSpark® Self-Publishing
© Ingram Content Group

**The Winner's Manual: Take Control of Your Life**
How to Ditch the Quick Fixes and Finally Produce Results That Last!

Bobby Lynch

*Cover Photo by Kewan Harrison*
*Website: 1010pro.com*
*Cover Design by Rob W.*
*Website: fiverr.com/cal5086*

**ISBN**
*Paperback: 978-1-7343329-7-1*

*For Dad. Until we meet again...*

*Love,*

*Bobby, Mom, and Ryan*

# Disclaimer

*Weight loss and muscle gain results will vary depending on the individual. Specific results are not guaranteed.*

Causes of being overweight or obese vary from person to person. Whether genetic or environmental, it should be noted that food intake, rates of metabolism, levels of exercise, and physical exertion vary from person to person. This means that weight loss and muscle gain will also vary from person to person. No individual result should be seen as typical.

The information, including but not limited to text, graphics, images, and other material, contained in this book is for educational purposes only. The content is not intended in any way as a substitute for professional medical advice, diagnosis, or treatment. Always seek the advice of your physician or other qualified healthcare provider with any questions you may have regarding a medical condition or treatment, and before undertaking a new weight loss program, diet, or exercise training regimen. Never disregard professional medical advice, or delay in seeking it because of something you have read in this book.

These statements have not been evaluated by the Food and Drug Administration.

Furthermore, by reading this book, you acknowledge that weight training, resistance training, cardiovascular conditioning, and other physical activities can be dangerous and could lead to potential injury or death. Any injuries, including death that result from training while using the Plant Strength Coaching program included in this book are because

## Commitment & Consistency

*The difference between those who see results and those who stay the same.*

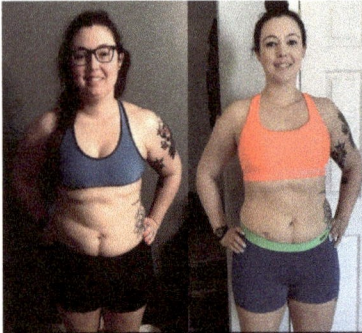
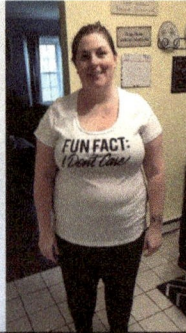
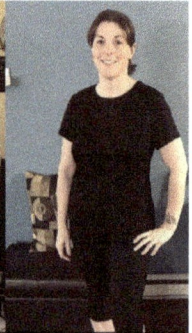

BEFORE AFTER BEFORE AFTER

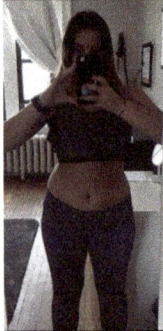
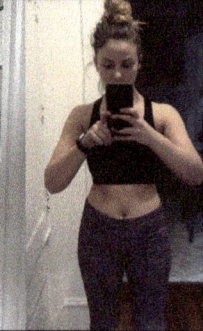
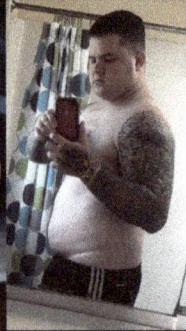
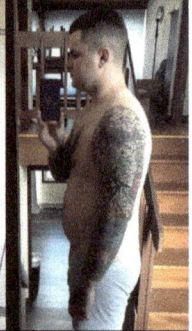

BEFORE AFTER BEFORE AFTER

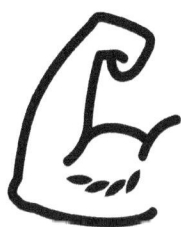

# Contents

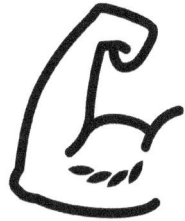

# Introduction

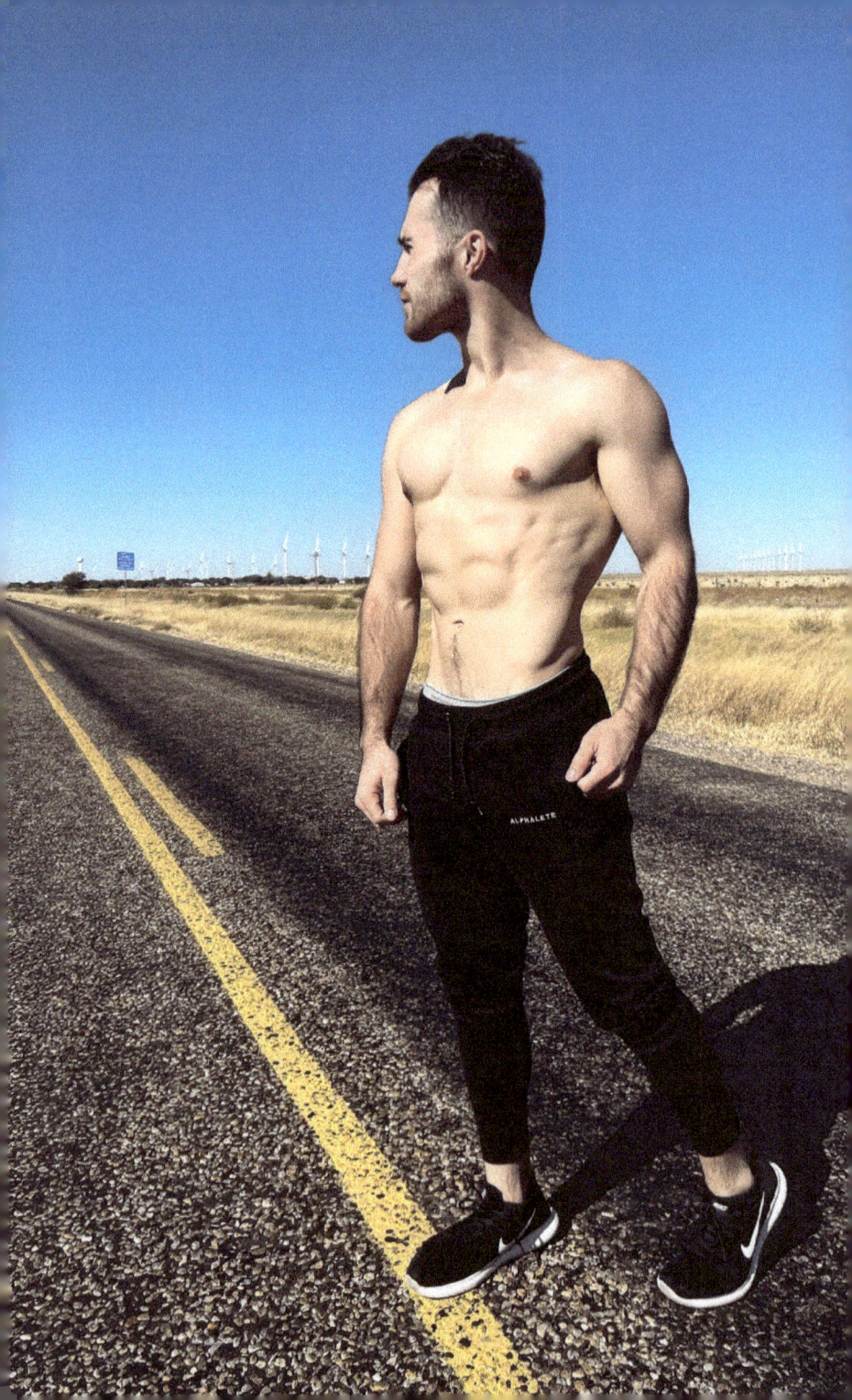

# My Journey into the Fitness Industry

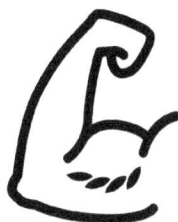

It's a funny story how I realized that this was my calling, and it all started with an ad on craigslist. Before we get into that, though, let me give you a little background about myself.

Ever since I was little, I've always lived an active life. When I was seven years old, I started playing tackle football, and I immediately fell in love with the sport. It wasn't until 16 years later that I played my final season at Union College. Along with football, I also played soccer, basketball, and baseball as a child. I started snowboarding when I was nine and got into paintball at 11.

My introduction to fitness came at a pretty young age. I first started working with a personal trainer at the Mystic YMCA also at age nine, and then after two years transitioned to Advantage Personal Training.

The winter following my freshman high school football season was when weight training became a serious deal. As I started to lift more and more, it became more than just preparing for the next year to me. It became a *lifestyle!*

Fast forward to November 2016, after I graduated from Union with a degree in Economics, I did what every other recent grad does at the time and started applying for as many jobs as possible within my field. I sent out cover letter after cover letter, resume after resume, hoping that one place would call me for an interview for a job that I likely wouldn't stay at for very long, but I'd be taking because it'd make me money and was *"something to do."*

But because the market was (and still is) saturated, which makes finding a job take forever, I went on craigslist looking for odd jobs around town to make money while I waited patiently for a callback.

Not long after logging on, I came across an ad posted by a lady named Suzanne (who's now a great friend of mine) that was six days old saying, *"In need of a personal trainer. I'm about 50 pounds overweight, and I could use someone to come to my house a couple times a week for coaching."*

Me being me, I replied to it, of course, saying, *"Still in need of a trainer?"* And, to my luck, she did!

We exchanged numbers and then scheduled a consultation. During our discussion, I explained to Suzanne that, although I wasn't officially certified, I was very confident I could help her. I've always had a passion for fitness, and I've practically had a running personal-training internship for the majority of my life while growing up at Advantage; not to mention all the professional coaching that I also received while playing football in college.

She liked what I had to say and hired me right there. We then scheduled our first week of workouts, and I returned a few days later for our first session. After what felt like the quickest 60 minutes ever, that's when it hit me; *this is what I wanted to do!*

Although I excelled in school, and for the longest time thought I was going to follow the corporate path and get a job on Wall Street, I've always had an entrepreneurial spirit and the desire to build my own business. And after leaving my first ever personal training session and thinking to myself, *"this is work?"*; what better company could I start than one in an industry I'm so deeply passionate about?

Not only could I take my love for fitness and nutrition and turn it into a career, but I'd also be bettering the lives of the people I was gifted to coach. *What more could I ask for!?*

I quickly enrolled in the **National Academy of Sports Medicine Personal Training Certification Program,** and the rest is history.

I do what I love each and every day, and I couldn't be happier with my life decision. I'm thankful for the opportunity to work with all the unique individuals that I work with daily and hopefully, one day, I'll get to work with you too!

**My ultimate goal is to affect positive change in as many lives that I possibly can: humans, animals, and our planet alike. With this book, I aim to do just that!**

*The Winner's Manual* **isn't a quick-fix diet plan** that promises you fast results, which ultimately disappear equally as fast once you start eating normally again.

**It'll teach you *everything* you need to know to *get in your best shape* and *stay in your best shape* for the *rest of your life.*** And do so in a cruelty-free way by eating food that tastes amazing and benefits not only your health but also the animals and our environment.

**It'll show you how to:**
- Build a **strong mind, body, and spirit.**
- Find **balance with your personal fitness and nutrition.**

- Finally *produce results that last!*

**I couldn't be prouder of this book, and I guarantee you'll love every page!**

If you have any questions, you may contact me directly at **bobby@plantstrength.com.** And yes, this is my actual email. As in, *I'll be the one who replies.* If you don't believe me, try it out for yourself. ;)

May your health forever prosper,

Bobby

**Part 1**

# Mindset

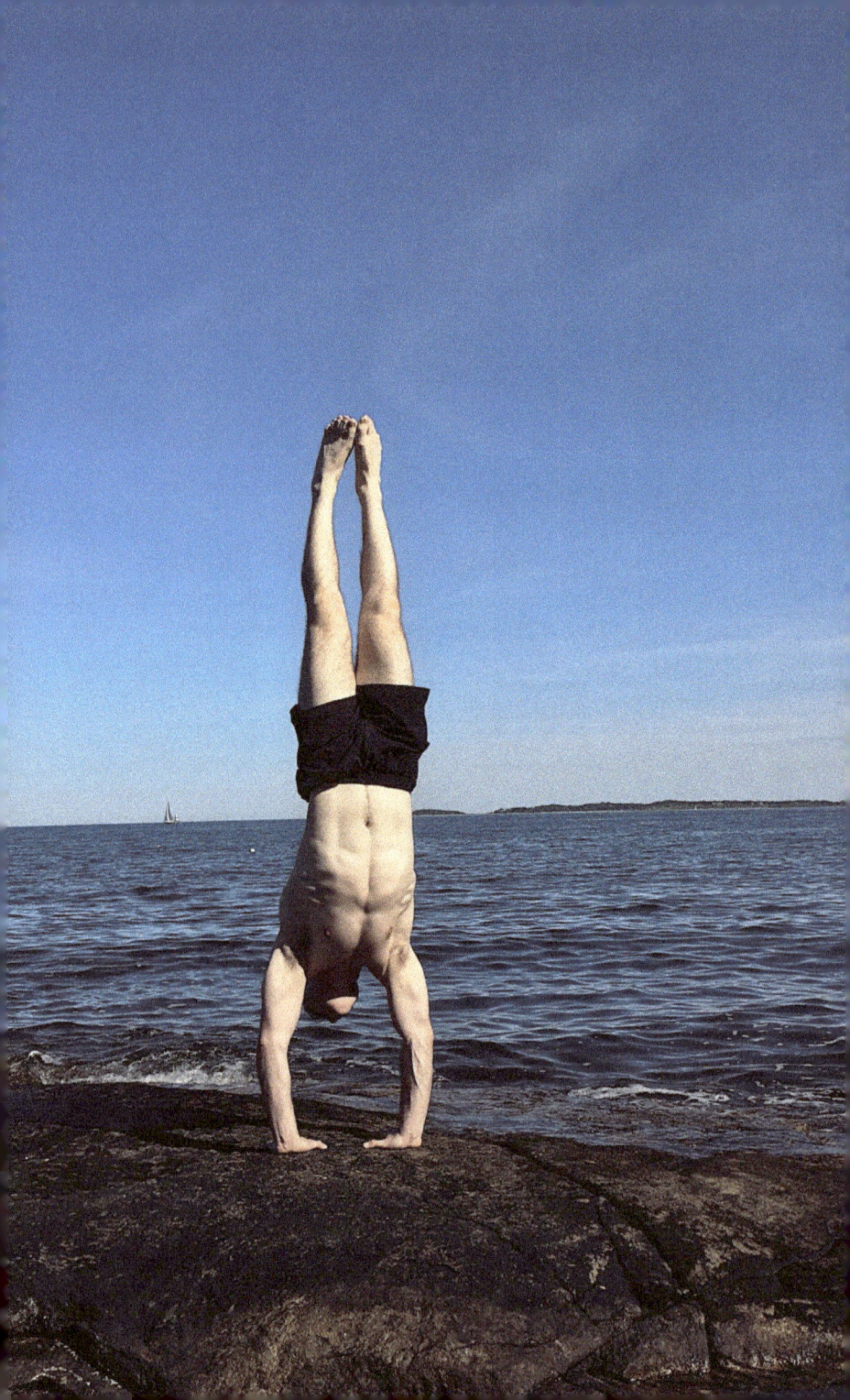

**1.1**

# Closed vs. Growth Thinking

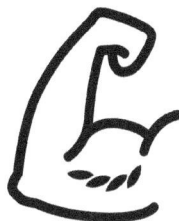

*"There is only one thing that makes a dream impossible to achieve: the fear of failure."*

*– The Alchemist* (Paulo Coelho)

**Before you can truly make *lasting* changes in your life, *you must first get your mind right.***

When people fail, it's usually for one (or all) of the following reasons:

1. Their mindset was closed and negative versus open and positive.
2. They either didn't start or gave up along the way because they feared *"failing."*
3. They didn't know their *"why."*

To better define what I mean by failing, **I mean *never* achieving what you set out to achieve–*ever.*** I don't mean making mistakes or having setbacks because you'll make and have many, and Plan A rarely works out, anyway.

However, **what will make the biggest difference in you learning from your mistakes, overcoming your setbacks, and accomplishing your goals is your *mindset!***

The idea of mindset was first discovered by Stanford University psychologist, Carol Dweck, and she says that mindset takes one of two forms:
- **Closed** (Fixed)
- **Open** (Growth)

| FIXED MINDSET | | GROWTH MINDSET |
|---|---|---|
| • SOMETHING YOU'RE BORN WITH<br>• FIXED | SKILLS | • COME FROM HARD WORK.<br>• CAN ALWAYS IMPROVE |
| • SOMETHING TO AVOID<br>• COULD REVEAL LACK OF SKILL<br>• TEND TO GIVE UP EASILY | CHALLENGES | • SHOULD BE EMBRACED<br>• AN OPPORTUNITY TO GROW.<br>• MORE PERSISTANT |
| • UNNECESSARY<br>• SOMETHING YOU DO WHEN YOU ARE NOT GOOD ENOUGH. | EFFORT | • ESSENTIAL<br>• A PATH TO MASTERY |
| • GET DEFENSIVE<br>• TAKE IT PERSONAL | FEEDBACK | • USEFUL<br>• SOMETHING TO LEARN FROM<br>• IDENTIFY AREAS TO IMPROVE |
| • BLAME OTHERS<br>• GET DISCOURAGED | SETBACKS | • USE AS A WAKE-UP CALL TO WORK HARDER NEXT TIME. |

[19]

When one has a **closed mindset,** he or she believes that their basic abilities, intelligence, and talent are *fixed* traits that cannot be changed. They feel they have no control over their situation, and only those born with *"talent"* will achieve success, and it'll come without effort. They shy away from challenges and typically get angry or defensive in the face of criticism. [22]

When one has an **open mindset,** he or she believes that their basic abilities, knowledge, and talent can be developed through dedication and hard work; and natural intelligence and talent are just starting points. They have a love for learning and *growth.* They embrace challenges with resiliency and welcome criticism with open arms because they know it'll only make them better. [22]

I used to have a closed mindset, and I remember clear as day when it was first pointed out to me. I was 14 years old, and it was during a workout at Advantage Personal Training with the owner, Greg Drab, and (now retired) NFL defensive lineman of 10 years for the San Diego Chargers, Jacques Cesaire **(@jacques.cesaire74).**

Every summer, Jacques would come from San Diego, CA to Mystic, CT, during July so that he could train at Advantage with Greg in preparation for the season.

In the summer going into my freshman year of high school, I was fortunate enough to have the opportunity to work out with Jacques, as he invited me to join in on a few workouts with him. During our workouts, Jacques would always talk to me about this concept of mindset and closed versus growth thinking. He explained it to me just as I described it above, and then one day in the middle of our workout, he told me that I had a closed mindset.

I remember standing there, in the small room off the side of the main lobby to the gym, and thinking to myself, *"Is he being serious? There's no way I have a closed mindset. He's got to be kidding me!"* I was so taken aback and had to do my best not to show how defensive I was. But, lo and behold, *he was right.*

Although I had always been a hard worker growing up (my work ethic instilled in me by my dad), *I hated criticism.* I would get so defensive over anything somebody said that went against what I was doing, had to say or what I believed, and I'd take everything to heart. And if I didn't achieve something, instead of taking ownership for my failure, I would blame it on the fact that I wasn't *"this,"* I wasn't *"that,"* the other person got *"lucky;" "blah, blah, blah..."*

The fact of the matter was, my mindset was closed. I always wanted to impress everyone and *"look my best."* I feared stepping out of my comfort zone for new challenges because I feared failure.

But what Jacques told me, which I'll never forget, was, *"Don't look at failure as failure. Instead, treat every 'failure' as an opportunity to learn"*–a chance to get better and grow. What a difference that statement has made.

**Thank you, Jacques.**

**1.2**

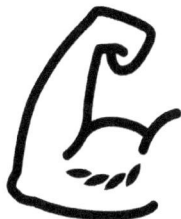

# Look for the Positives

**No matter what you're trying to accomplish, you'll *always* have setbacks along the way.** Unless you're born into wealth or fame, no path to success is ever a straight line. You'll mess up. You'll make mistakes. We're human, that's what we do. But it's about how you look at your mistakes that makes all the difference.

**To transform your mind, you must *look for the positives* in every situation.**

Instead of worrying about the fact that you *"failed,"* take a deep breath, assess what went wrong, and then formulate a new plan for going forward. Take away from your *"failure"* the fact that you now know information that you didn't know prior, and that you should try something new, or slightly different the next time.

And if you try your new plan and *"fail"* again, it's all good; it's a part of the process. Re-assess, reformulate, and give it another go.

For two years, I had been trying to present my "Health, Wealth, Balance" presentation on managing a busy schedule, working out, eating well, and staying in shape as a working professional at Union College, my alma mater.

Ideally, my target audience was the senior athletes about to graduate, as I was an athlete myself, and I know just how hard it can be once you enter the working world to stay in shape. I've seen a number of my athlete friends quickly fall out of shape upon leaving school and working full time because they no longer have the strict training regimen of their sport and they can't *"out train"* their bad diets anymore.

To set this presentation up, I had many meetings with the career center director and members of the wellness center, both over the phone and in-person (mind you, Union is over 180 miles from where I live), and initially, things were repeatedly denied for one reason or another.

Finally, in the spring of 2018, my presentation was approved, and I went up for ReUnion weekend (a big family-and-alumni gathering on campus held every year in May) to present.

Guess how many people were at that presentation.

Six–the Career Center Director and his wife, the Assistant Director of the Counseling Center for Health Promotion, my former strength & conditioning coach, one student, and my brother. Seven–if I count myself. Eight–if you count the janitor working in the basketball center where my presentation was held.

Now, I could have easily chalked this up to be one big *"failure."* I could have gotten angry that flyers weren't actually made and posted until only a day prior; and no campus-event email was sent out to students or faculty, which is usually done for events and presentations like these.

I could have blamed Bob (the Career Center Director) or Amanda (the Assistant Director of the Counseling Center for Health Promotion) for *"not trying hard enough"* and left campus upset and with bridges burned.

Well, not only would that have been the dumbest thing ever, the truth is, Bob and Amanda *actually worked very hard* to try and get this going. They did what they could within *their* power, but the fact is, if I wanted to present to the athletes, I should have gone right to the people who have direct control over them and their coaches—the athletic director and the head athletic trainer.

Moreover, because Amanda, Bob, and Dan (the Head Strength & Conditioning Coach) all saw my presentation and got to see first-hand exactly what I brought to the table, it gave me even more credibility for when I actually went directly to Jim (the Athletic Director) and Cheryl (the Head Athletic Trainer), because they could now reference Amanda, Bob, and Dan.

And guess what? The following year, I presented to an audience of almost 30! But not on ReUnion weekend this time. Instead, on the weekend following because, as Cheryl pointed out, ReUnion is not a great weekend for presentations because of all the other events already taking place. More information learned that I otherwise wouldn't have known if I hadn't *"failed"* the first time.

Now, one might say, 30 people isn't a lot. Which, when compared to an audience size of say 500, yes, 30 is quite small. But the previous year I had only presented to an audience of six; meaning in 2019, I increased my audience size by five times! *Perspective.* ;)

On top of that, I made many connections that day, which will only lead to more doors opening down the road.

**Always look for the *positives* in every situation and *embrace losing!*** Welcome it with open arms! Understand that **you're going to lose *way***

*more* **than you actually win.** But once you do finally win, you'll realize that **all of your** *"failures"* **were** *100% worth it!*

Every *"overnight success"* was predicated by years of hard work and *many "failures."* And those *"failures"* helped shape those people to become who they are today.

If your dream is something you can't stop thinking about, then not going for it or giving up because you fear failing is stupid, as you'll live your whole life in regret.

**You only have one life, so give it all you've got and** *don't fear failure!* **You've already won!** You're alive, and you're human–more than many people (and creatures) can say.

# Overcoming Limiting Beliefs

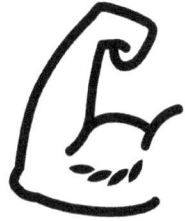

Before you're capable of realizing the positivity in your external failures, **you must first find it within *yourself*,** and that starts with the conversation going on in your head. If you're always telling yourself, *"I can't do something," "I don't deserve success,"* and *"he/she/they will think I'm a loser if I fail";* then you're already defeated. This is a fixed mindset, which creates an internal monologue that's focused on judging. [22]

Instead, you must switch that monologue to one of constructive action and positivity.

- *"I can do this; it'll just take time."*
- *"I deserve success, but it'll take hard work."*
- *"It doesn't matter what anybody thinks, I'm pursuing my goals because doing so makes **me** happy."*

**Your reality is whatever *you* make it. What you continually tell yourself will ultimately come true.** If you have a fixed mindset, that's okay. Remember, I used to too. But if you follow the steps in the next chapter, taken directly from Carol Dweck herself, you can change your mindset and finally get on your path of growth and success.

**1.4**

# Transforming Your Mind

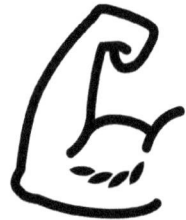

## 1. Learn to Hear Your Fixed Mindset "Voice"

As you approach a challenge:

That voice might say to you, *"Are you sure you can do it? Maybe you don't have the talent. What if you fail—you'll be a failure. People will laugh at you for thinking you had talent. If you don't try, you can protect yourself and keep your dignity."*

As you hit a setback:

The voice might say, *"This would have been easy if you really had talent. See, I told you it was a risk. Now you've gone and shown the world how limited you are. It's not too late to back out, make excuses, and try to regain your dignity."*

As you face criticism:

You might hear yourself say, *"It's not my fault. It was something or someone else's fault."* You might feel yourself getting angry at the person who is giving you feedback. *"Who do they think they are? I'll put them in their place."* Even if it's specific, constructive feedback, you might still be hearing them say, *"I'm really disappointed in you. I thought you were capable, but now I see you're not."* [21]

## 2. Recognize You Have a Choice

How you interpret challenges, setbacks, and criticism is your choice. You can perceive them with a fixed mindset as signs that your fixed talents or abilities are lacking. **Or you can view them with a growth mindset as signs that you need to ramp up your strategies and effort, stretch yourself, and expand your abilities.** It's up to you.

So, as you face challenges, criticism, and setbacks, listen to the fixed mindset voice and... [21]

## 3. Talk with a Growth Mindset Voice Instead

As you approach a challenge:
- The **Fixed-Mindset** says, *"Are you sure you can do it? Maybe you don't have the talent."*
- The **Growth-Mindset** answers, *"I'm not sure I can do it now, but I think I can learn to with time and effort."*
- **Fixed Mindset:** *"What if you fail—you'll be a failure."*
- **Growth Mindset:** *"All successful people had many failures along the way."*
- **Fixed Mindset:** *"If you don't try, you can protect yourself and keep your dignity."*
- **Growth Mindset:** *"If I don't try, I automatically fail. Where's the dignity in that?"*

As you hit a setback:
- **Fixed Mindset:** *"This would have been easy if you really had talent."*
- **Growth Mindset:** *"That is so wrong. Basketball wasn't easy for Michael Jordan, and science wasn't easy for Thomas Edison. They had a passion and put in tons of effort."*

As you face criticism:
- **Fixed Mindset:** *"It's not my fault. It was something or someone else's fault."*
- **Growth Mindset:** *"If I don't take responsibility, I can't fix it. Let me listen–however painful it is–and learn whatever I can."*

Then... [21]

## 4. Take the Growth Mindset Action

Over time, which voice you heed becomes your choice. Whether you:
- Take on challenges wholeheartedly.
- Learn from your setbacks and try again.
- Listen to criticism constructively and act.

**All of this is now in your hands.**

Practice hearing both voices and then acting on the growth mindset. See how you can make it work for you. [21]

**1.5**

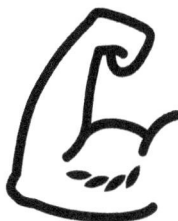

# Positive Mantras

What helps me tremendously with maintaining my growth mindset is reciting positive mantras, both in my head and out loud–all of which are custom for me based on my personal goals and the life I want to create.

**Some of my positive mantras include:**
- I AM successful.
- I have EVERYTHING I need to be happy.
- No obstacle is too big to overcome.
- *The Winner's Manual* is a HUGE SUCCESS.
- Plant Strength is a HUGE SUCCESS.
- I am positively affecting millions of lives worldwide.
- I am traveling the world as I please.
- I have set my family up to live financially free.

No matter your goals or for what you want your life to be like, **your positive mantras should be written and recited in the *present* tense as if you've already achieved everything you desire.**

**Remember, *your reality is whatever you make it*. What you continually tell yourself will ultimately come true.** If you always speak as if you've already accomplished your goals and built your dream life, then that's what will happen if you match your actions to it!

Write your positive mantras down and make multiple copies. Place one at your bedside, one on your fridge, and one on your desk in your office. Repeat your mantras to yourself at least once every day. I spend the last five minutes of every meditation session (meditation,[1] something I practice daily) repeating positive mantras in my head.

I do the same thing if I ever feel anxious, overwhelmed, or start doubting myself. I pause, take a deep breath, and recognize that what I'm feeling is *only temporary.* I then begin reciting my positive mantras, usually starting with, *"No obstacle is too big to overcome."* And just as fast as those negative thoughts and feelings crept into my mind, they quickly start fading away.

Try reciting your mantras every night before going to bed, first thing in the morning after you wake up, or both. Get in the habit of repeating them every day and watch how your dreams will slowly start manifesting in front of you.

> *"When you want something, all the universe conspires to help you achieve it."*
>
> – *The Alchemist* (Paulo Coelho)

---

[1] See "Meditation," page 227.

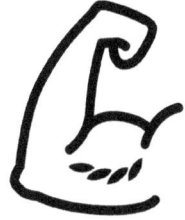

# Finding Your *"Why"*

Writing positive mantras also means writing down your goals, and with every goal must be a reason for wanting to achieve it–your *"why."*

This *"why"* is the driving force behind your motivation because when it starts to wane (as motivation usually comes and goes), reminding yourself of the root reasons for why you're doing something will keep you committed to actually doing it.

For example, my most significant reason going vegan (more on this next section) was because I don't believe in the suffering and killing of innocent living beings. At first, however, when I was only vegetarian and still consuming eggs and dairy products, I wasn't fully connected to my *"why."*

But after seeing many documentaries and eye-opening social media posts, I learned that this suffering and killing takes place in *all* animal agriculture, not just the meat industry. Once I knew that, it became easy to look at the ingredients of foods I used to enjoy, see that they contained meat, dairy, eggs, or some other animal product, and then turn them down without a second thought.

How? ***Because I fully connected to my "why" and continuously remind myself of it every day.***

The same thing goes if you're trying to lose weight. If your goal is to lose 30 pounds, is it merely because you want to lose 30 pounds for the sake of doing so, or is it something deeper? Such as you want to:

- Lose those pounds to lower your blood pressure.
- Relieve the pain in your knees that you experience daily from carrying extra weight.
- Get back to playing with your kids regularly, which you haven't been able to do in a while because being overweight drains your energy and causes you to quickly lose your breath.
- All of the above.

**Really digging deep and finding your *"whys"* will be the difference-maker when you hit obstacles, have setbacks, or feel like giving up.** Once you know them, like your positive mantras, write down your goals with their accompanying *"whys."* Make multiple copies and carry one around with you. When negative temptation sets in, simply pull out your goals list and remind yourself for why you're set on achieving them.

At first, it might be difficult to resist your temptations. But like with anything, it takes time. The more you do this, the easier it'll become and soon enough, saying no to things that detract from your success will become a piece of cake—*and cake tastes good!*

**1.7**

# Banish ALL Doubt

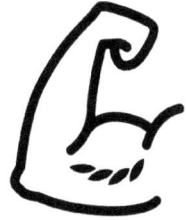

> *"There is only one thing that makes a dream impossible to achieve: the fear of failure."*

> – *The Alchemist* (Paulo Coelho)

I started this section with the quote above, and I repeat it again here because it couldn't be more accurate. **The only thing holding you back from your success is** *the fear of failure.*

But is failing really that fearful? Think about it. What's the worst that can happen? You set a goal, and things don't go as planned–again, *they usually never do;* or you don't accomplish your goal by the date for which you set to achieve it.

*So what!* At least you tried. Because **what's the alternative?** Not trying? Never going for it. Living your life in regret because you were too afraid to give your dreams a shot for fear of things not working out. *That's silly!*

**We're all going to die one day.** Do you really think that when it's all said and done, you're going to look back and think, *"Man, I'm glad I was fearful and didn't pursue my dreams,"* or *"I'm glad that I didn't even try to achieve the one thing that I couldn't stop thinking about"?* I don't think so.

**The key to life is** *happiness.* **Doing whatever is going to make you insanely happy day-in-and-day-out.** What good does it do to doubt yourself in achieving something that's going to bring an abundance of happiness to your life? *It doesn't!*

> *"The only true obstacle lies within the doubt itself–and all doubt lies within your own thoughts ... [It's] a waste of energy and interferes with your natural ability to create the abundance and wealth that is your birthright."* [15]

You already have everything you need to be happy, and you already know everything necessary to be successful. But to realize that success, you must **trust yourself** and **banish ALL doubt.**

A lot easier said than done, of course. But here's how you do it:

1. **Imagine what your life would be like if you were to achieve your goals.**
   - How much better would it be?
   - How would you feel?
   - What would you be doing?
2. **Now imagine the alternative if you were to doubt yourself and never attempt them or give up along the way.**
   - How much worse would your life be?
   - How would you feel?
   - What would you be doing?
3. **Every time you start doubting yourself,** *think of the alternative.* Soon enough, you'll realize just how silly all of that doubt is.

**1.8**

# WIN THE DAY

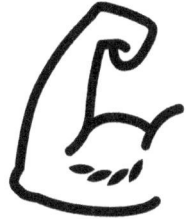

Lastly, and most importantly, *WIN THE DAY!*

**Don't think too far ahead.** Have your end destination in mind but realize that, to go from A to Z, you must first stop at B, C, D, and every other letter in between.

**Take small steps.** Create little sub-goals necessary to achieving your big one. **Be patient, *win each and every day,* and soon enough you'll realize your success. It'll just take time.**

# Part 2

# Why Vegan?

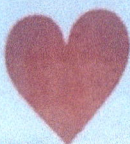

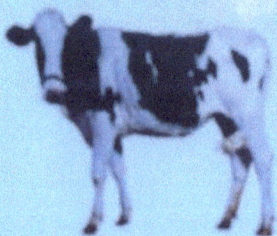

**2.1**

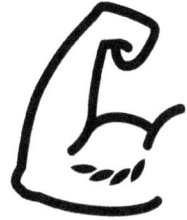

# The Root of All Evil

I find it amazing that as a country we spend the most money on healthcare in the entire world, but we have the sickest people. **In 2017, Americans spent $3.5 trillion on healthcare alone.** [18] **The GDP (Gross Domestic Product) for the United Kingdom in 2018 was only $2.62 trillion.** [10]

In simple terms, GDP represents the sum of all revenue made by every industry in a country. **This means that the United States' healthcare system by itself makes more money than all the money made from every industry in the fifth richest country in the world.** Let that sink in.

On top of that, **we eat the most meat (aside from Iceland); yet we have some of the highest rates of cancer, diabetes, heart disease, and obesity, and close to the lowest longevity of any developed nation.** [20] The average American consumes some sort of meat or animal product three times per day, and it's usually the centerpiece of the meal.

The average American also suffers from cancer or some sort of chronic disease. In fact, **one in every three American women and one in every two American men will be diagnosed with cancer at some point in his or her life,** [20] and together, *one in every four will die from their diagnosis.* [4]

And the saddest part about this is that most people think this is normal. Even doctors. To the majority of the population, the belief is that *"disease just happens."*

> *"Cancer isn't the result of a systematic disequilibrium–it's an invasive monster. Heart disease isn't the logical outcome of excess fat and chronic inflammation–it's genetic bad luck. Diabetes isn't the product of a diet that consistently raises your blood sugars–it's just what happens to some people."* [20]

As if humans are frail creatures destined to die slow and horrible deaths from equally horrific diseases. But the fact of the matter is, *we're not!* **Our health is a direct result of what we put in (and on) our bodies every day.**

No one wants to believe that though. No one wants to accept that the cause of most (if not all) of their health issues is the result of all the cheeseburgers, sausages, and steak dinners they've been consuming their whole life. No one wants to be told when going to the doctor that *they* are actually the cause to their own problems. They'd rather just take a pill or have surgery and continue with their poor habits because cancer and disease are *"inevitable."*

They're *"here for a good time, not a long time"* is something I've been told by far too many people. But how can you have a *"good"* time if you're not in good health? If you're always sick, lethargic, and overweight; how can your life be enjoyable? Because at least you get to eat your bacon? Come on now.

I never wanted to believe all of this, too. I grew up eating meat, drinking milk, and eating eggs. My family (mom, dad, brother, and I) would go through two dozen eggs and seven gallons of milk a week; not to mention the pounds of meat.

Just a few years ago, a typical day of eating for me looked like the following:

- Five eggs and a cup of egg whites scrambled with some veggies and cheese for breakfast
- Yogurt and granola for a mid-morning snack
- Grilled chicken wrap with a salad for lunch
- Beef jerky or a protein bar for an afternoon snack
- Two scoops of whey protein in a shake after my workout
- More chicken, or steak, pork, or fish with potatoes or rice and veggies for dinner
- Ice cream or cookies for dessert (when desired)

I'd always make sure to have vegetables with each of my three main meals; *but, holy cow, was that a lot of animal protein!* Pun fully intended (lol). It's no wonder my cholesterol was almost 200! I was eating upwards of 250-300 grams of protein a day, pretty much all of it being animal protein, which also comes packed with tons of saturated fat and cholesterol.

And it's not like I was out-of-shape at the time either. That sample meal plan above was an average day of eating for me while playing football in college when I weighed an average of 170-180 pounds at 10-15% body fat depending on the time of year.

Now that I'm vegan, my weight nor body-fat percentage hasn't changed much, and neither has my activity level. However, the last time I had my cholesterol checked, it was only 137–*a huge difference!*

But still, to most people, this is *"healthy"* eating. *"The more animal protein, the better!"* Right? Or so we're always told. That's all you hear nowadays. Protein this. Protein that. It's the first thing everyone asks me when I tell them I'm vegan: *"Where do you get your protein?"*

**Little do they realize (as I once didn't either) that virtually all plant foods have protein and contrary to popular belief, *almost every one of them contains all essential amino acids.***

But, somehow, we've been led to believe that the only way to build muscle and avoid protein deficiency is by eating pounds of meat and eggs and drinking whey protein shakes–*which couldn't be further from the truth!*

Let me ask you, do I look protein deficient? *I didn't think so.*

Then why is this necessity for animal protein all that we hear about? Because that's how they want it; *"they"* referring to the colossally rich, immensely powerful animal agriculture industry worth hundreds of billions of dollars that dominates our market and controls our country.

It's crazy (and scary) how much control they have over us. Don't believe me?

**The dairy industry spends at least *$50 million* each year, promoting its products in public schools. The meat and dairy industries together spend upwards of *$140 million* each year lobbying Congress. They also spend over *$550 million* promoting animal products through federal USDA commodity checkoff programs [4]–** catchy advertisements such as the *"Beef, It's What's for Dinner®"*

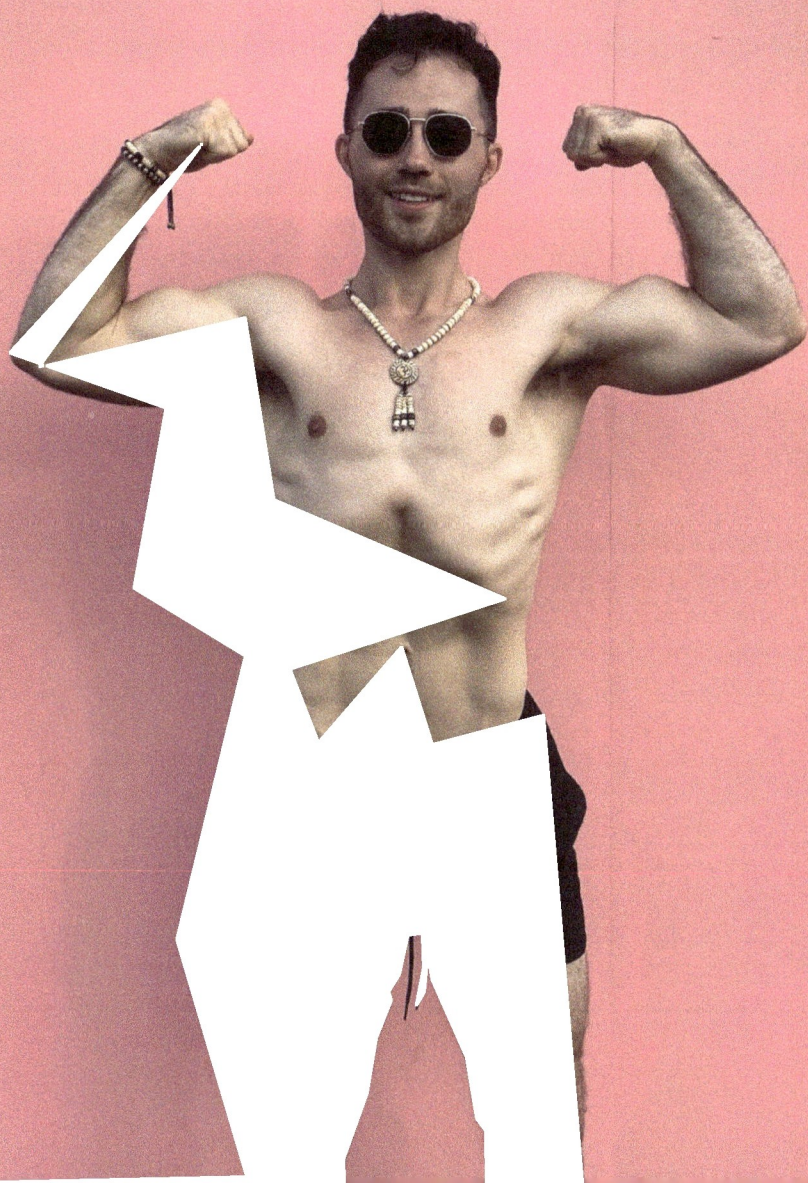

And that's not even the half of it.

**The American Heart Association is partnered with the Texas Beef Council. Tyson Foods is partnered with both the American Heart Association and the American Cancer Society, and Dannon and Bumble Bee Seafoods are both sponsors of the American Diabetes Association.** [4]

On top of that, **all of these organizations accept millions of dollars indonations from pharmaceutical companies; and the pharmaceutical industry just so happens to sell** *80%* **of all antibiotics made in the United States to animal agriculture because there are** *at least 450 drugs* **known to be administered to these animals.** [4]

Starting to see the connections? We live in a money-hungry society dominated by a healthcare system that supposedly has our *"best"* interests in mind; yet never seems to fix the problem, just treat the symptoms. **But if we actually attacked the root cause of these diseases and, instead, worked on** *preventing* **them before they ever happened; there wouldn't be a need for doctors to prescribe all the pills, medicines, stomach stapling, heart transplants, scraping of plaque from arteries, or excruciatingly painful treatments of chemoradiation.**

People would instead be healthy and thriving. The fact of the matter is though, people can't be healthy. We need to be sick because, without the demand for these overtly expensive commodities, billions of dollars in revenue would be lost; and that's just unacceptable.

**So, even though animal protein has been shown time and again to promote cancer, diabetes, and heart disease; and the World Health**

Organization has actually *classified bacon and sausage as carcinogenic to humans*–meaning *they're known to cause cancer;* these organizations still promote the consumption of meat and animal products as *"healthy."* In fact, *the American Cancer Society even recommends eating processed turkey and canned meats!* [4]

Have you ever heard of the saying, *"money is the root of all evil"?* It very much applies.

# Health Effects of Animal Protein

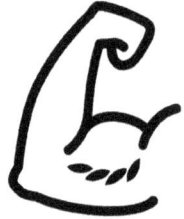

It's time to shift gears and dig deeper into the effects of animal protein on the body, and we're going to start with the big one.

## Cancer

Cancer is something that sits very close to me, as my dad passed in August 2015 from it. He was only 55 at the time. His cancer was a rare form called GIST (Gastrointestinal Stromal Tumors), and the strain he had was very aggressive. It made him so weak that during the last month of his life, he was unable to walk on his own. I had to either wheel him in a wheelchair or carry him chest-to-chest with his arms draped over my shoulders to help him get from room-to-room around the house.

Ultimately the disease took over his body and consumed him. It changed his appearance so much that we had him cremated after he passed because he wouldn't have been recognizable to people who hadn't seen him in a while.

Now you may be wondering how my dad got this disease in the first place, and to be honest, so am I. He lived a very active and healthy life. He loved running, and he'd run five to six miles a day, on top of lifting weights three to four days each week. He'd have two pieces of fruit every day with lunch and a salad almost every night with dinner. He never ate fast food or drank soda, and always drank plenty of water. His alcohol consumption was very moderate and consisted of a glass of red wine when we went out on the weekends for dinner, and a light beer here or there during the week. He never used drugs, and he and my mom had quit smoking long before I was born.

But again, as a family, we ate a lot of meat and drank a lot of milk. The typical rotation of our family dinners was:

- Baked or grilled chicken
- Pork chops
- Burgers and hot dogs
- Steak
- Spaghetti with meatballs and sausage
- Mac and cheese
- Take out
- Dinner at a restaurant–which usually included a variation of one of the above

One of my dad's favorite restaurant meals was a sirloin steak cooked medium-rare.

Unfortunately, however, data from the EPIC (European Prospective Investigation into Cancer and Nutrition) study in which hundreds of Europe's top scientists followed 521,000 people from ten European countries, concluded that **the more red and processed meat one eats, the higher their chance of developing stomach and colon cancer.** [20] That was exactly the type of cancer my dad had, and we ate red meat on average two to three times a week.

Not only did the EPIC study conclude this, but an Australian study following 37,000 people for nine years also showed that **as the consumption of red and processed meat went up, so did the rates of rectal cancer.** [20]

The NIH-AARP (National Institutes of Health and the American Association of Retired Persons) study, which looked at 500,000 men and women between the ages of 50 and 71 for ten years, had similar findings, as well, as it showed that **high red and processed meat consumption was significantly associated with cancers of the colon, esophagus, and liver.** [20] And it doesn't stop there.

These studies, among many others following hundreds of thousands of people over many years–like **the Multiethnic Cohort Study of Hawaii, the Health Professionals Follow-Up Study, the Nurses' Health Study, and meta-analyses of multiple studies–all show associations between meat and other types of cancer: breast, lung, pancreatic, and renal-cell alike.** [20]

Why is this? Research isn't yet entirely conclusive. However, many things point to highly likely causes. Like **heme-iron and IGF-1** (Insulin-Like Growth Factor 1), for example.

**Heme-iron** is a form of iron only found in animal products. Although still theory, it's thought to produce unstable N-nitroso compounds (NOC) in the body, which have been linked to high risks of gastrointestinal cancer by one of the EPIC studies. The study found that **the more heme-iron one consumes, the more NOC found in their stool and the higher their risk for rectal cancer.** [20]

**IGF-1** is a human growth hormone that our bodies produce naturally, but whose circulation increases with the consumption of animal protein. Now, you're probably wondering, why would high levels of a growth hormone, one that our bodies produce naturally, be a bad thing? That's because **IGF-1 promotes the growth of cells and inhibits their death.**

As babies and children, we have higher levels of IGF-1 because we need it to grow. But once we've reached adulthood and have finished growing, **if we already have cancer cells forming within our body (it takes years for cancer to grow large enough to be detectable), then increasing levels of our circulating IGF-1 will only accelerate the cancerous cell growth, while also preventing its death.** [20]

**And what significantly increases your levels of IGF-1?** *Animal protein.* This doesn't mean just meat. It means eggs and dairy too.

> *"Most female cows are routinely injected with growth hormone to get them to produce milk as fast as possible. This IGF-1 seeps into their milk, which is then absorbed into our bodies when we drink it (even when pasteurized)."* [20]

Then we must drink hormone-free organic milk, right?

Nope. This milk also contains high levels of IGF-1, as dairy milk was designed to transform a 400-pound baby calf into a 2,000-pound mammal in as little time possible. [20]

Another probable cause is the chemicals that form in meat and animal products when cooked at high temperatures known as **HCAs** (Heterocyclic Amines) that are already involved in many cancers. [20]

On top of that, **you also have all the chemicals pumped into the animals during their raising and slaughter,** which come from the hormones and antibiotics used to make them rapidly grow and keep them *"healthy";* and from the pesticides in the food they ingest. Once the animals are killed, those chemicals don't just magically disappear; they're locked into the meat. So, **when you consume that meat, you also consume all of those chemicals with it.** [20]

On the opposite end of the spectrum, **diets heavy in meat and animal products (Atkins, keto, and paleo, for example) also reduce the number of protective bacteria (phytochemicals) found in the body because the people following them consume relatively low amounts of fruit and vegetables compared to vegans and vegetarians.**

**Phytochemicals** are *biologically active compounds found only in plants, such as carotenoids, fiber, flavonoids, specific vitamins, and many other minerals;* **which have been shown to significantly decrease the risk of cancer when consumed in high amounts.**

**But it's not just high amounts of phytonutrients that significantly decrease cancer risk, it's that combined with** *an avoidance of the toxins found in meat, dairy, and eggs.*

The Health Professionals Follow-Up Study of 48,000 men showed exactly this by holding not only fruit and vegetable consumption equal; but also saturated fat, total fat, and animal fat. This means that the only variance was found in the amount of dietary animal protein that was eaten. The conclusion? **The more animal protein one consumed, the higher the risk for colon cancer.** [20]

In fact, the EPIC-Oxford study found that, overall, **vegetarians have an 11% lower risk for cancer than meat-eaters, and vegans have an even lower risk at 19%.** [31]

So, just eating your fruit and veggies isn't enough. **If you want to reduce your risk for cancer, then you must also** *reduce (preferably eliminate) your consumption of animal protein, too.* This makes sense because, although my dad ate plenty of fruit and vegetables daily, he still died of cancer.

What's to say though that my dad's cancer was caused only by the animal protein he ate? If that was the case, then why wouldn't everyone his age, who consumes the same amount of meat and animal products (or more) throughout their lifetime, be dying of the same cancer? That's a great question. Again, the evidence isn't 100% conclusive that *all* animal protein causes cancer, and it's easy to say correlation doesn't equal causation. But:

> *"There are many great long-term studies that draw attention to the link between animal protein and cancer...[and] if there is a correlation in multiple studies from multiple parts of the world, and these correlations have been put through rigorous analysis, then you better believe there is something to the correlation."* [20]

**And remember, it's already been proven that *canned and processed meats do cause cancer.***

To bring attention back to my dad though, it's still unknown as to what caused his disease. Being informed, after the fact, that the government office building he had worked in for years was found to be ridden with asbestos; and that there had already been several people from that building who died of cancer; it's likely that was the trigger to start his cancerous cell growth. But even if it was, his regular consumption of meat and animal products surely didn't do any good with deterring further growth; and it's highly likely that it only made things worse.

## Diabetes

Second, we have diabetes. More specifically, I'm talking type 2 diabetes (when the body overproduces insulin), also commonly known as adult-onset diabetes.

According to the Centers for Disease Control and Prevention, as of 2015, **close to 10% of the U.S. population suffers from type 2 diabetes, and close to 30% is pre-diabetic; meaning, they're insulin-resistant and on the way to becoming full-blown diabetic.** [17] And if you were to ask almost everyone in the U.S. (diabetics, pre-diabetics, and non-diabetics alike) what the cause of diabetes is, my guess is nearly 99% would blame carbs and sugar.

However, the reality is that **carbs and sugar are *not* the cause of diabetes. *They're an aftereffect*–a symptom of becoming insulin-resistant, which is greatly exacerbated by refined carbs (like table sugar) that cause large spikes in your insulin.**

**The *real* cause of diabetes is intramyocellular fat:** *the fat stored within the muscle tissue in your body that blocks the muscle's ability to uptake glucose, which then causes insulin resistance.* Let me explain.

**As humans, our primary source of fuel is sugar (glucose). Every cell in our body utilizes it for energy. The average adult brain, alone, needs 130 grams per day to function correctly.** This is why when carbs are digested, no matter the source (whether brown rice, sweet potato, or table sugar), almost all are broken down into the simple sugar, glucose. Fruit will break down into the other simple sugar, fructose.

Once dietary carbs are digested and the sugar enters your bloodstream, your pancreas secretes **insulin:** *a storage hormone used to shuttle nutrients to your cells.* If not used immediately for energy, the extra sugar will be stored in your muscles and liver as glycogen. Glucose will primarily store in the muscles, while fructose in the liver.

**A healthy adult can store between 300-600 grams of glycogen in their muscle tissue and another 80-100 grams in their liver–a total**

of 380-700 grams (or 1,520-2,800 calories) worth of carb storage at once.

How well your muscles uptake this sugar depends on your cells' ability to develop new insulin receptors. When someone suffers from diabetes or insulin resistance, it means their development of new insulin receptors is poor. What inhibits this ability? *Intramyocellular fat.* [20]

When someone eats meat, they're consuming protein and fat. **Contrary to popular belief, not only carbs but protein and fat also raise insulin levels too, as insulin is used to shuttle *all* nutrients to your cells. In fact, according to the Insulin Index of Foods, *beef actually raises insulin more than pasta* with an insulin score of 51% compared to only 40%, respectively.** [26]

**The difference between meat and carbs, however, is that the meat itself, as well as the saturated fat that comes with it, causes inflammation in the body, which damages muscle cells and results in fat accumulation in the muscle tissue.** [20]

**The cause of this inflammation is due to several factors, one of which is known as acidosis.** When your body's pH is acidic, calcium is leached from your bones and muscles to neutralize this acidity. However, when calcium is taken from your muscle cells to buffer the acid, it causes muscle wasting and leads to fat deposition within. [20]

**Meat also causes inflammation from the endotoxins in it that are produced by harmful bacteria, like salmonella.** Although these bacteria are killed when cooked at high enough temperatures, the endotoxins stay planted inside. Thus, when the meat is consumed, the saturated fat causes the endotoxins to be absorbed into the body, and your immune system responds through inflammation. [20]

Therefore, **when overeating and consuming excess calories in the form of meat and saturated fat, you gain weight through a build-up of fat, much of which will be stored in your muscle tissue from inflammation.** This intramyocellular fat then inhibits the muscle's ability to properly uptake glucose in the cell *(aka, insulin resistance),* making the pancreas think it didn't produce enough insulin to get the job done and signaling it to produce more.

**The more intramyocellular fat you have, the more insulin resistant you become, and the more insulin your pancreas needs to produce. Perpetuate this cycle of excess body fat and insulin resistance for years, and sooner or later, you end up with diabetes.** Once you have diabetes or are pre-diabetic, high intakes of simple carbs then result in even higher levels of insulin, worsened insulin sensitivity, and more body fat stored if you're continuously overeating.

So again, **carbs and sugar are *not* the cause of diabetes.** They're a symptom. **The *real* culprit is large quantities of fat stored within the muscle tissue (intramyocellular fat) caused by overeating and exacerbated by inflammation from high consumption of meat and saturated fat.** [20] The exact reason for why you never see someone of a healthy weight with type 2 diabetes. Only those who are severely overweight have it.

In terms of studies, unfortunately, there hasn't been any large randomized control trials yet that specifically compare a plant-based diet devoid of animal protein to a high-protein animal product diet, like Atkins or Paleo, with regards to diabetes.

However, when you look at population studies around the world (the EPIC Study, Adventist Health Study, Nurses' Health Study, Health Professionals Follow-Up Study, Women's Health Initiative), the prevailing trend is that **the more animal protein and the less fruit and vegetables consumed, the more incidence of diabetes. Whereas populations who consume the majority of their calories in the form of fruit, veggies, and starches all experience much lower diabetic rates.** [20]

In fact, the EPIC study found that **"glucose and fructose consumption was actually correlated with *less* diabetes… [and by replacing] just 5% of the saturated fats in your diet with fructose, you reduce your risk of developing diabetes by a whopping 30%."** [20]

I actually consulted with a lady for coaching once who had severe type 2 diabetes. She was 80 years old, stood 5'1" tall, and weighed over 240 pounds. Her doctor's prescribed diet plan to help *"manage"* her diabetes, which I've copied and pasted directly from my consultation notes below, was:

- **Breakfast:** Three small sausages, scrambled eggs, and toast
- **Lunch:** Tuna fish sandwich on two slices of whole wheat bread with chips and tea
- **Dinner:** Four ounces of fish or hamburger with baked potato, green beans, and asparagus
- **Snacks:** Ice cream and peanut butter crackers

After going through her long list of medications, she tells me her doctor (the same one who prescribed the diet plan above) said *"she'll be on those medications for life and will never get off them."*

**However, she also then proceeded to tell me that her church pastor used to also have type 2 diabetes too, but he now no longer does; nor does he take any more medication. When I asked her how he cured himself, she told me he said, and I quote, *"I stopped eating meat and went fully vegan."* Need I say more?**

## Heart Disease

Next up, we have the number one single cause of death in America. Can anyone guess it? That's right: *heart disease.*

Research from the American Heart Association's AHA 2018 Heart Disease and Stroke Statistics report estimates that **one million Americans will have a heart attack or die from coronary heart disease this year alone, and currently, 16.5 million U.S. adults (age 20 or older) are living with this deadly disease.** And those numbers are barely a fraction of the amount that suffers from **hypertension** *(high blood pressure).* Current estimates are that over 100 million Americans suffer from high blood pressure, which is 46% of the U.S. adult population. [3]

Yes, you read that right. *More than 100 million Americans* **suffer from a direct cause of our number one killer, heart disease, as well as stroke and kidney disease.** And these numbers are just for the U.S. **It's estimated that over** *one billion* **people suffer from hypertension worldwide.** [20]

For those of you unfamiliar with blood pressure and what yours should be, normal blood pressure is lower than 120/80 mmHg (millimeters of Mercury).

- The top number represents **your systolic blood pressure:** *the pressure in your blood vessels when your heart beats.*
- The bottom number represents your **diastolic blood pressure:** *the pressure in your blood vessels between beats.*

Old guidelines used to say that a blood pressure reading of 140/90 mmHg or above was classified as hypertension. However, the AHA's new guidelines as of November 2017 classify that **anything 130/80 mmHg or above is considered high blood pressure.**

## Blood Pressure Categories

American Heart Association | American Stroke Association®

| BLOOD PRESSURE CATEGORY | SYSTOLIC mm Hg (upper number) | | DIASTOLIC mm Hg (lower number) |
|---|---|---|---|
| NORMAL | LESS THAN 120 | and | LESS THAN 80 |
| ELEVATED | 120 – 129 | and | LESS THAN 80 |
| HIGH BLOOD PRESSURE (HYPERTENSION) STAGE 1 | 130 – 139 | or | 80 – 89 |
| HIGH BLOOD PRESSURE (HYPERTENSION) STAGE 2 | 140 OR HIGHER | or | 90 OR HIGHER |
| HYPERTENSIVE CRISIS (consult your doctor immediately) | HIGHER THAN 180 | and/or | HIGHER THAN 120 |

©American Heart Association

**heart.org/bplevels**

With a number like 100 million, you'd think that medical efforts would be full force into lowering blood pressure; and indeed, they are. But of course, through the use of pharmaceuticals that only manage the symptoms, *not fix the problem*–which just so happens to be the American diet high in meat and saturated fat.

Unlike with cancer and diabetes where the research isn't yet entirely conclusive (although very much points to animal protein being the culprit); **there have been numerous studies of various sample sizes conducted in many different countries over short and long timespans alike that all clearly show diets high in meat and saturated fat *cause* both hypertension and heart disease.** [20] Two of which I previously discussed (the Adventist Health Study and the EPIC study) that have both followed thousands to hundreds of thousands of people for many years.

In the Adventist Health Study, researchers compared *"healthy"* meat eaters to vegetarians and vegans (whose diet was devoid of animal protein), and they found that **the more animal protein consumed, the higher one's overall blood pressure and the greater their risk for developing heart disease.** [20]

In the EPIC study, specifically the Oxford branch, researchers also compared a population of *"healthier than average"* meat eaters (whose meat consumption was much lower than the average intake) to an *"unhealthy"* group of vegetarians (due to their low fiber intake and calcium and vitamin B_{12} deficiencies). Their findings?

"Despite this seemingly unfair comparison, **the unhealthy vegetarians still had significantly lower rates of hypertension than the healthy meat-eaters... [and a] statistically significant 30% reduction in the risk of developing heart disease by eliminating animal protein from the diet.**" [20]

The INTER-MAP study (the INTERnational Study of Macronutrients and Micronutrients and Blood Pressure), one of the best-regarded hypertension studies, followed over 4,600 people while looking at the relationship between diet and blood pressure and found that **"vegetable protein had a significant blood-pressure-lowering effect."** [20]

But it's not just population studies that show this. Many other randomized control studies, which have tested the effects of only increasing fruit, to only soy, to eliminating meat completely, have all shown that **adopting a vegan or vegetarian diet lowers blood pressure and the risk for heart disease.** In fact, "a meta-analysis of randomized trials looking at replacing animal protein with soy protein... [showed] **soy protein significantly reduces LDL cholesterol and**

**triglycerides, two known risk factors for heart disease."** [20] Why is this?

**It could be due to several reasons, the first of which is inflammation**–a leading cause in the formation of heart disease. And as we just discussed, diets high in animal protein and saturated fat heavily inflame the body.

**Second, we have the cholesterol that comes packed with animal protein,** which tightens blood vessels and restricts blood flow to vital organs. Restricted blood flow then leads to high blood pressure and over time, heart disease.

**Third, is heme-iron (only found in animal protein),** which causes oxidation and is directly associated with the development of heart disease.

**Finally, we have the abundance of protective phytonutrients (found only in plants)** that you obtain through a diet high in fruit and vegetables (antioxidants, fiber, flavonoids, vitamins, minerals) that combined with zero animal protein intake, decrease inflammation, cholesterol, and blood pressure and thereby reduce the risk of heart disease. [20]

So, in short, **if you want to lower your blood pressure and decrease your chance of developing heart disease,** *then skip the meat and eat more fruit and veggies!*

## Obesity

Lastly, we have the effect of animal protein on obesity–a condition that as of 2015 affects 40% of American adults (over 93 million to be exact), and is a precursor to many diseases: cancer, diabetes, and heart disease to name a few. [16]

Obesity is classified as having a **Body-Mass Index (BMI)** of 30, or higher and is calculated by dividing your weight in kilograms (kg) by your height in meters squared. For example, at 67 inches and 170 pounds, my BMI is 26.6.

## BMI Calculation

- 1 in. = 0.025 m
- 67 in. = 1.702 m
- 1 lb. = 0.454 kg
- 170 lbs. × 0.454 kg = 77.111 kg
- **BMI:** $77.111 \div 1.702^2 = 26.6193$

Technically, this BMI classifies me as *"overweight,"* as a BMI of 25-29.9 is considered to be. But, clearly, I'm not overweight. At 170 pounds, I'm roughly 12% body fat with a 31-inch waist. Why is my BMI considered *"overweight"* then?

### BMI Chart

| Classification | BMI |
|---|---|
| Underweight | < 18.5 |
| Normal Weight | 18.5-24.9 |
| Overweight | 25-29.9 |
| **Obese** | **30-34.9** |
| **Clinically Obese** | **35-39.9** |
| **Morbidly Obese** | **> 40** |

[11]

When the BMI measure was created in the 1830s by Lambert Adolphe Jacques Quetelet, a Belgian astronomer, mathematician, statistician, and

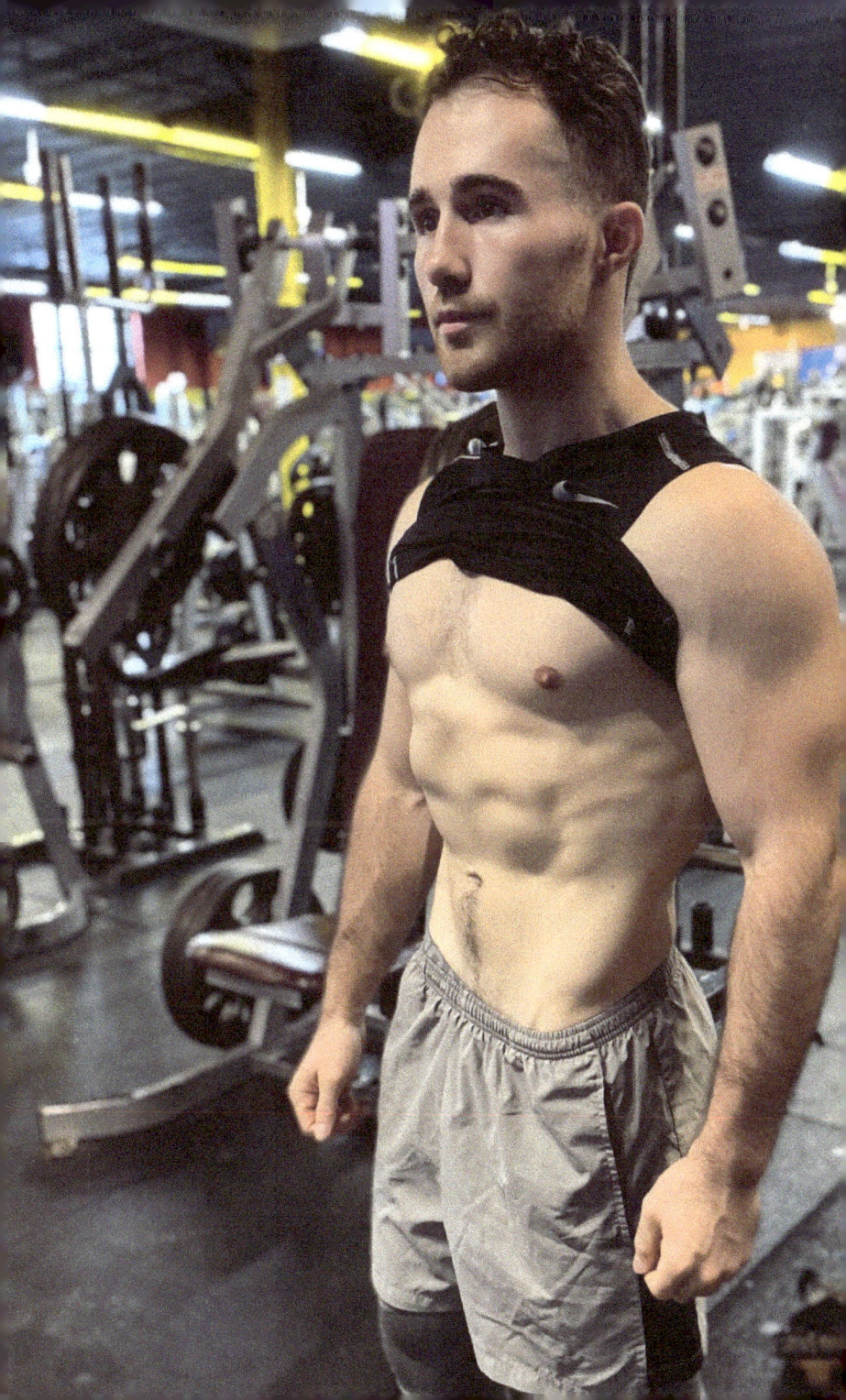

sociologist, [32] it was designed to measure people with a relatively average **lean body mass:** *everything that comprises your weight (bone, muscles, organs, water, etc.) minus your fat.* [11]

Thus, athletes, bodybuilders, and other people who have higher than average amounts of muscle will have a greater than average lean body mass and a higher weight overall. This will then skew classifications as to what you actually are (underweight, healthy weight, overweight, obese) because BMI is only a measure of your total weight divided by your height. It doesn't account for muscle mass or body-fat percentage.

Nonetheless, for the average person in America, obesity is a big problem (no pun intended); and our diet heavy in meat and animal products is only making things worse.

In simple terms, **what causes weight gain is *overeating.*** A major theme this book revolves around (which you'll see starting next section) is *calories in versus calories burned.* All food is comprised of energy (calories). Thus:

- If you're taking in less energy (calories) than you're burning, then you'll lose weight.
- If you're taking in the same, then you'll maintain your weight.
- If you're taking in more than you're burning, then you'll gain weight.

So, technically, **you could eat only McDonald's every day and lose weight as long as you're eating fewer calories than you're burning.** Mark Haub, a professor of Nutrition at Kansas State, proved this concept by losing 27 pounds on his junk-food diet.[2] [20]

---

[2] See "Fad Diets," page 145.

The opposite is also true in that you can gain weight by only eating plain tofu and rice if you're consistently eating more than you're burning. However, in both cases, it'll be tough to accomplish the respective goal due to the caloric density of the foods.

Meat and animal products, especially processed ones from fast food restaurants like McDonald's, are calorically dense. Compared to their plant-food counterparts, the number of calories per weight is very high. For example, 100 grams of cooked beef sirloin, the *"healthiest"* beef for you (and I use *"healthiest"* very loosely), yields over 210 calories. Your standard McDonald's cheeseburger yields over 260. One hundred grams of cooked broccoli, however, contains only 35. [1]

One hundred grams is less than four ounces. According to predictions from the USDA, the average meat eater consumed 10 ounces of red meat and poultry each day in 2018. [20] Ten ounces of beef sirloin has over 600 calories, and sirloin is the leanest cut of beef.

### Beef vs. Broccoli Calorie & Macro Comparison

| Food | Calories | Fat | Sat. Fat | Cholesterol | Fiber | Protein |
|---|---|---|---|---|---|---|
| Broccoli | 100 | 1 | 9 | 9 | 10.5 | 7 |
| Beef Sirloin | 600 | 28 | 10.5 | 250.5 | 0 | 83 |
| Ground Beef (85/15) | 710 | 44 | 16.5 | 255 | 0 | 73.5 |
| McDonald's Cheeseburger | 745 | 34 | 12.5 | 99 | 3 | 37 |
| Ground Beef (70/30) | 775 | 52 | 21 | 232.5 | 0 | 72 |

*Nutritional info represents "cooked" data from **acaloriecounter.com**. Serving Size = 10 oz.*

Being generous and assuming the average person consumes 85/15 (%) (lean/fat) ground beef (when in reality it's likely 70/30 because 70/30 is cheaper), 10 ounces of cooked ground beef has over 700 calories! Ten ounces of cooked broccoli has less than 100, and also no cholesterol, no saturated fat, and far more micronutrients and phytochemicals.

Now a meat eater's counterargument to this would be, *"Well look at all the protein in beef. That's why there are so many calories. Plus, protein is good for you. The more, the better!"*

I actually laughed out loud while writing this because I used to say that exact same thing when I used to eat meat. Yes, a lot of the calories in beef come from protein. But other than beef sirloin, the majority of the calories in all other cuts of beef come from fat. And more protein beyond what you need doesn't equate to better, either. Especially if it's animal protein.

**Protein provides only four calories per gram, whereas fat provides nine. Thus, over 55% of the calories in 85/15 ground beef** *actually come from fat*, **and 60% for 70/30 beef–and a lot of this fat is saturated fat.**

The RDA recommends that men have no more than 30 grams of saturated fat per day, and women no more than 20 grams. **If you're a woman and consume just 10 ounces of 70/30 ground beef, then you've already surpassed your saturated fat limit for the day,** *and that's just from your beef consumption alone.*

Add in the cheese, eggs, milk, and other meat you've also likely consumed during the day, and you could easily be over double your daily limit by day's end; not to mention your caloric maintenance requirement. And that's not even accounting for all the fat and calories from the oil you've likely cooked with, as well.

People already have a problem with overeating and pushing past fullness. Now factor in that a lot of what they're overeating is high in calories, low in volume, and devoid of fiber and tons of other essential nutrients, it's no wonder so many people in America are sick and overweight. **All we hear is** *"protein, protein, protein,"* **and** *"more, more, more!"* **Yet the more we consume, the sicker and more obese we seem to become.**

The picture below is an excellent illustration of caloric density and everything I just talked about and is the precise reason for why it's so easy to overeat on an animal protein-heavy diet, but nearly impossible to do so on a plant-based one.

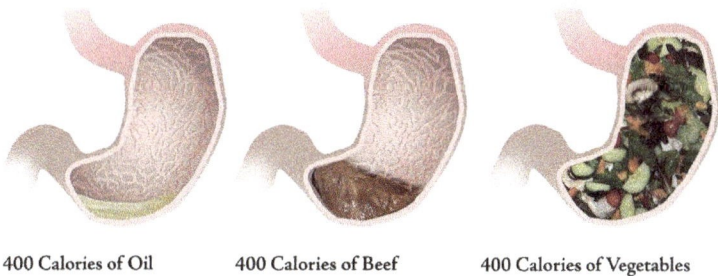

400 Calories of Oil          400 Calories of Beef          400 Calories of Vegetables

© 2012 Julieanna Hever, MS, RD, CPT • www.PlantBasedDietitian.com
Illustration by Sherri Nestorowich • www.sherrinest.wix.com/art

Furthermore, the second Adventist Health Study conducted between 2002-2006 that looked at the prevalence of diet on body weight and type 2 diabetes, which comprised of over 22,000 men and 38,000 women, showed that **the mean BMI of vegans was only 23.6, whereas for meat eaters it was 28.8. This makes the average meat eater overweight**

**and nearly obese.** It also showed that **less than 3% of vegans suffered from type 2 diabetes, but the incidences in meat eaters were almost 8%.** [14]

On top of that, if you look at the diets of the people from the longest-lived cultures in the world (the one's author and National Geographic explorer, Dan Buettner, calls the *"Blue Zones"*), meat and fish consumption averages less than 5% of the diet; dairy less than 9%; and egg consumption a whopping 1%. This means that 85% or more of their food intake is fruit, grains, legumes, and vegetables. [13]

**The five Blue Zones include:**
- Ikaria, Greece
- Okinawa, Japan
- Sardinia, Italy
- Loma Linda, California
- Nicoya Peninsula, Costa Rica

In terms of macronutrients, 60-80% of their diets are comprised of carbs. **For example, the diet of the Okinawans of Japan (who have the most centennial women–the most women to have lived into their 100s), consists of *80% carbs,* 10% fat, and 10% protein. Their staple food source is the Japanese sweet potato. And meat is consumed *at most* once to twice a month on special occasions and in servings of *only* three to four ounces at a time.** [13]

Circling back to my statement that more protein beyond what's necessary isn't better for you; the current U.S. government RDA (recommended daily allowance) for protein is 0.8 grams per kilogram of body weight (BW). Again, that's **0.8 grams *per kilogram* of BW, not per pound.**

I emphasize this because when you ask almost anybody in the fitness industry what the recommendation for protein intake per day is (including the proclaimed *"fitness pros"*), most everyone will say one gram per pound of BW (something I also used to recommend before I knew better), which, for most people, is much more than they actually need. Some even go as far as recommending two to three grams per pound of bodyweight. Did somebody say, *kidney disease!?*

- The recommendation of 0.8 grams per kilogram is for the average sedentary adult.
- If you live a more active weekend-warrior type life, then upwards of one gram per kilogram will suffice.
- For athletes who train more regularly (like those in high school and college), up to 1.2 grams per kilogram is suitable.
- And at the very most, elite endurance or strength training athletes (bodybuilders, football players, marathoners, and powerlifters) will benefit from upwards of 1.8-2.3 grams per kilogram of BW in protein per day.
  - But again, this is the *absolute most* one will ever need to build and maintain the muscle necessary for their elite sport; and is in grams *per kilogram* of BW, not per pound. [7]

Thus, as a 170-pound athlete, at the *very most* I need 178 grams of protein per day. And that's assuming I had a very active day and I'm eating in a deficit. If I stay between 77 grams and 178 grams of protein on average, I'll be perfectly fine. And again, clearly, I'm not protein deficient.[3]

- 1 kg = 2.2 lbs.
- 170 lbs. ÷ 2.2 kg = 77.23 kg (1 g/kg)
- 77.23 kg × 2.3 g/kg = 177.63 g

---

[3] For more on calculating your protein needs, see "Calculating Your Macros," page 163.

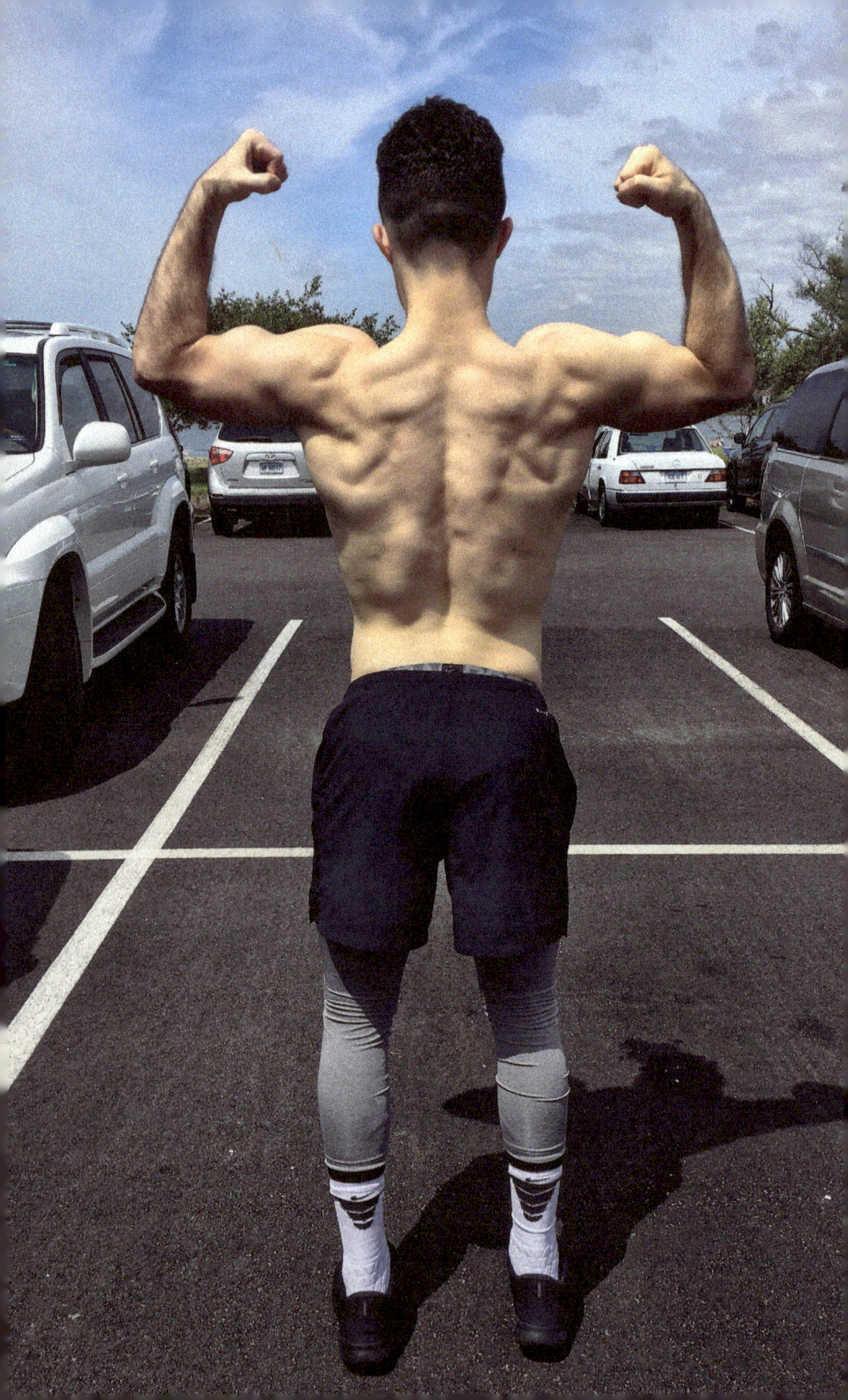

Consuming far more than my uppermost requirement is not only unnecessary, it's also unhealthy if done for a prolonged time.

First, unlike with carbohydrates and fat, where we have large storage capacities for them, we have limited storage for protein. Thus, **excess protein consumed beyond what you need is ultimately converted into glucose for use as energy or excreted as waste through your urine.**

Second, **consuming more protein than what's necessary puts extra stress on the kidneys to rid the body of the high levels of nitrogen waste produced through protein metabolism.** If this constant build-up of nitrogen waste is drawn out over long periods of time, it puts you at risk for the development of kidney disease and is extremely detrimental if you already have it. [20]

Lastly, the source of protein matters. Animal protein (meat, dairy, and eggs), as already shown, contributes to a host of deadly diseases: cancer, diabetes, heart disease, and many more. **If the majority of your protein intake already comes from meat and animal products, and on top of that you're consuming way more protein than you actually need, you're only increasing your chances for many health problems down the road.** [20]

So, in short, **what causes obesity isn't one particular macronutrient or food. Obesity is due to a lifetime of habitually overeating.**

However, **because meat and animal products are calorically dense, often high in saturated fat, and devoid of fiber, they easily contribute to overeating and weight gain, which leads to obesity over time.**

Moreover, the adverse health effects of animal protein that usually take years to show themselves will ultimately show if the majority of your daily protein intake consistently comes from animal protein.

**If you want to live a long, happy, and healthy life, then skip the meat, drop the dairy, forgo the eggs, and start filling your body with plants! Trust me, *it'll be one of the best decisions you ever make!***

# Ethical Effects of Animal Agriculture

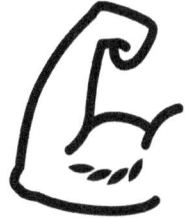

*"When I see cages crammed with chickens from battery farms thrown on trucks like bundles of trash, I see, with the eyes of my soul, the Umschlagplatz (where Jews were forced onto trains leaving for the death camps). When I go to a restaurant and see people devouring meat, I feel sick. I see a holocaust on their plates."*

– Georges Metanomski, a Holocaust survivor who fought in the Warsaw Ghetto Uprising

The biggest reason for why I went vegan was because of ethics. I've always been an animal lover, and really a lover of all life (insects included); I always escort spiders and other bugs out of my house and never kill them. I'm not a malicious person by any means and could never imagine intentionally killing another living being, especially to eat its dead body afterward.

Growing up, however, the connection between what I was eating and what it used to be was never there. Yes, I always knew that I was eating chicken, turkey, steak, and ham; and that meat came from a chicken, turkey, cow, or pig. But what was on my plate was just that: *"chicken," "turkey," "steak,"* or *"ham."* It was food, and those were the names for it. As if it were any other food like broccoli, peanuts, potatoes, rice; you name it.

All I saw was the well-prepared, well-seasoned, and aromatic piece of meat—the final product, never the process. Which is why the connection to the fact that that meat actually came from sentient creatures who were once living, breathing, had families, felt fear, and had the desire to live like you and I was never entirely made because their slaughter was never witnessed, nor was the life of suffering that they lived. And that's how the industry wants it.

If more people saw the truth behind what goes on during the production of meat and all animal products, and then took the time to fully empathize with these beautiful creatures, without a doubt many more people would be vegan; and the animal agriculture industry would lose billions of dollars. But of course, to maintain their power and profits, the industry spends hundreds of millions of dollars each year to keep their processes hidden from the public eye and to make it *seem* as if the animals are living *"happy"* lives.

- Ads with cows grazing in open fields of luscious green grass beneath vibrant blue skies.
- Slogans like *"cage-free," "free-range,"* and *"grass-fed"* stamped on packages.
- People-like cartoon animals smiling and giving a thumbs up.
- Or merely the final product cooked and plated, and accompanied by a family laughing and enjoying themselves at their dinner table.

**The reality of it, though, is that there is neither happiness nor enjoyment in the animal agriculture industry.**

Unless raised on a small family farm, practically all meat, dairy, and eggs come from animals raised on factory farms or feedlots, where they're crammed into tiny cages, stalls, or boxes barely larger than their body and left sometimes standing knee-deep in their own feces. They never see the light of day, breathe fresh air, or move from that space during their lifetime until the day they're loaded onto trucks headed to the slaughterhouse.

**All animals within the industry are ultimately killed. Dairy cows and egg hens too. Once their bodies are used past their limits and they can no longer produce their byproducts, they're rounded up and shipped to be killed for meat.** And no, *they don't live happy lives either,* no matter how magnificent the deceitful slogans make it seem.

*"Cage-free"* simply means the chickens are raised without cages but doesn't refer to their living conditions. More often than not, cage-free chickens are housed by the thousands in large pens inside factory farms. Healthy, sick, and dead chickens alike all reside within the same area and are packed on top of one another with barely enough room to move.

*"Free-range"* is no better. This term is regulated by the USDA for use only with poultry produced for meat; but isn't for pigs, cattle, or egg-producing chickens, nor are the requirements strict at all. As long as the chickens have access to the outdoors each day for some time, even if it's just a few minutes, then eggs and poultry can be labeled as *"free-range."*

*"Grass-fed"* is probably the most misleading of them all, as most people confuse it with *"pasture-raised"* (something I used to confuse myself). Unlike *"pasture-raised,"* which means that the cattle spent some time outdoors on pasture, feeding on grass or forage; *"grass-fed"* simply means that the animal's primary food source after it's weaned comes from grass or forage, not from grain or corn. It doesn't refer to their living conditions. This doesn't make *"pasture-raised"* better though, as there are no government standards for this label; and, like *"free-range,"* the time spent outdoors is also unspecified.

Moreover, **none of these slogans mention the antibiotics used to keep the animals alive in their unsanitary conditions, or the hormones used to make them grow twice the size in half the time.** Unless clearly labeled as *"raised without antibiotics/hormones"* or *"no antibiotics/hormones administered,"* then one or both were used during their lifetime. [23]

**Furthermore, the cruelty in the treatment of the animals is unfathomable.**

To keep the animals confined in the tight spaces they live in, they're mutilated without anesthesia or pain relief. Dairy cows, pigs, and sheep have their tails cut off. Chickens are debeaked. Male cattle are dehorned. Male cattle and pigs are castrated. [9]

Dairy cows are repeatedly artificially inseminated (i.e., *raped*) because they need to stay pregnant to produce milk. Once they give birth, their babies are immediately stripped from them and sent to the veal industry to be locked in a box and then killed only four months later. **Male chickens born into the egg industry are macerated at a day old.** And any animal that shows resistance of any kind is beaten, stabbed, or electrocuted.

Once ready to be killed, the animals are packed onto trucks open to the elements and transported miles through all weather extremes, typically without food or water. The ones who make it alive to the slaughterhouse are then gassed to death, shot in the head, have their throats slit, or thrown into scalding hot water. [33]

**It's actually estimated that close to one million chickens each year are accidentally boiled or drowned alive.** [8] Your worst nightmare is a real-life hell for billions of animals. If you don't believe me, check out the documentaries **Dominion** and **Earthlings,** and you'll see first-hand what these creatures suffer through.

**Estimates are that over *55 billion* land and sea animals are killed annually just for U.S. consumption. That's over *150 million* animals per day! *PER DAY!*** [8] And that doesn't even include the estimated *63 billion* pounds of marine bycatch each year that are killed, as well. [12]

**Bycatch** is *the catch of non-target fish and ocean wildlife (seals, sea lions, dolphins, sharks, coral reef, etc.) including what is brought to port and discarded at sea.* **Estimates are that *40%* of all marine catch comes from bycatch.** [12]

To help put this into perspective, it's estimated that over 60 million people were killed in combat during WWII on all sides. Factor in another eight million exterminated by the Nazi regime and we're upwards of 70 million deaths over six years.

**In the next 24 hours, more than double that number of animals will be killed for food in the United States alone.** And over 25% of those animals will die for nothing, as an estimated 26.2% of U.S. retail meat gets discarded by stores or consumers (21.7% by consumers)–***fourteen billion* animals killed each year to, ultimately, be thrown away.** [8]

A great quote by 1978 Nobel Laureate, Isaac Bashevis Singer, goes as follows:

> *"Human beings see oppression vividly when they're the victims. Otherwise they victimize blindly and without a thought."*

It's easy to sit back and pretend like this stuff doesn't happen, but the truth is that *it does.* We need to collectively start trying to see things through the eyes of the victims. **If you don't believe in the suffering and killing of innocent living beings,** *then don't give your money to an evil industry that does!*

## 2.4

# Environmental Effects of Animal Agriculture

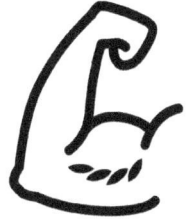

Not only is animal agriculture responsible for billions of deaths each year both directly and indirectly, but it's also causing the slow death of our planet.

One of the most significant and trending issues of today's time is climate change. The temperature of our planet is rising rapidly due to the rapid rise of greenhouse gases, which is slowly causing a host of adverse effects.

Before the start of the industrial revolution in the mid-1700s, atmospheric carbon dioxide ($CO_2$) sat on average at 280 parts per million (ppm). By 1950, it had risen to 310 ppm. Today it sits at 410 ppm, meaning in the last 70 years alone, it's increased 100 ppm! [30]

Why is this a bad thing, you may be wondering? Naturally, the Earth's levels of $CO_2$ will rise and fall over time with the coming and going of ice ages. However, they'll never rise as quickly as they recently have on their own.

**Life of today has adapted to live with low levels of $CO_2$. Dramatically increasing atmospheric levels wreaks havoc in so many ways:**
- Global warming
- Brutally hot summers
- Beyond freezing winters

- Ocean acidification
- Glacial melting
- Higher sea levels
- Species extinction

And more! [30]

When most people think of what's causing such high levels, they believe the leading cause is the burning of fossil fuels by factories, homes, and vehicles. **The real reason, however, is actually *animal agriculture.***

In a comprehensive study by the Worldwatch Institute, they found that **livestock and their byproducts (farts and manure) are responsible for 51% of all worldwide greenhouse gas emissions.** [27] **At least 32 million tons of $CO_2$ is their annual contribution.** [5]

But that doesn't account for the additional **13% contributed through the transportation of the animals to their slaughter, and then their meat to supermarkets**. Nor does it factor the other **18% contributed during their raising by emissions from factories, the production of feed, and the deforestation of land.** [5] Add those up and we're looking at **a combined total of *82%* of worldwide greenhouse gas emissions caused in some way by animal agriculture.**

It doesn't stop there, though. **Animal agriculture is also responsible for:**
- **Up to 91% of the Amazon rainforest destruction.**
  - Over 110 million rainforest acres cleared so far.
  - 1-2 acres cleared every second.
  - The extinction of up to 137 animal/insect species per day.
- **55% of U.S. water consumption (34-76 trillion gallons used annually).**

- **20-33% of all freshwater consumed worldwide.**
  - 2,500 gallons per pound of beef.
  - 1,000 gallons per gallon of milk.
  - 900 gallons per pound of cheese.
  - 660 gallons per hamburger.
  - 500 gallons per pound of eggs.
- **The use of 45% of Earth's total land.**
  - 2-5 acres per cow.
  - 1.5 acres necessary to produce only 375 pounds of meat per year compared to 37,000 pounds of vegetables.
- **3.5 trillion pounds of excrement produced every year in the U.S. alone.**
  - 130 times more than human waste.
- **2.7 trillion animals pulled from the ocean each year.**
  - 1:5, fish:bycatch ratio. Meaning, for every pound of fish caught, up to five pounds of unintended marine species are caught and discarded as **bycatch.**
  - 650,000 whales, dolphins and seals are killed every year by fishing vessels, and 40-50 million sharks are killed in fishing lines and nets. [5]

And these are just some of the numbers. **With our current farming of the oceans, it's estimated that they'll be *lifeless* by as early as 2048.** [35]

**Tyson, America's largest meat producer** *(and don't forget, a partner of both the American Heart Association and the American Cancer Society),* **dumps more toxic pollutants into our waterways than companies like ExxonMobil and Dow Chemical.**

> *"[In 2014], Tyson Foods, Inc. or its subsidiaries dumped more than 20 million pounds of pollution directly into our waterways... [and*

*this] figure only includes pollutants reported to U.S. EPA's Toxic Release Inventory and doesn't include pollution from factory farms raising livestock for Tyson." [39]*

In terms of food and water consumption, humans drink 5.2 billion gallons of water and eat 21 billion pounds of food throughout the world each day. **Cows alone drink 45 billion gallons of water and eat 135 billion pounds of food each day.** [5]

**We currently grow enough food to feed 10 billion people, yet worldwide, *over 800 million are classified as starving or malnourished.*** [2] In fact, *82%* of starving children live in countries where food is fed to animals that are then eaten by western countries. [5] Does that even make sense?

**We grow enough food to feed the world's entire population plus three billion more, *but close to one billion still go hungry.*** If not for that fact alone, we shouldn't be animal farming, not to mention the destruction it causes the planet.

**Animal agriculture is slowly destroying our home and the life within. If we don't start making drastic changes *now,* then our children and our children's children will greatly suffer from the effects of what we're doing.**

# The Benefits of a Vegan Diet

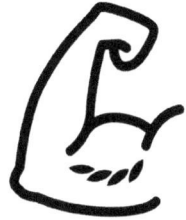

Now that we've looked at the host of adverse effects caused by animal protein and agriculture, let's look at the positive impact of a plant-based diet. We'll flow in the same order starting with our health.

## Health

Not consuming animal protein means you're also not consuming heme-iron nor HCA's, which have both been linked to or shown to be a direct cause of cancer.

Neither will you have high levels of circulating IGF-1 that greatly accelerate cancerous cell growth and prevent its death.

You also won't be ingesting the antibiotics and hormones pumped into the animals during their raising that stay locked within their meat once killed, which are also highly probable cancer causes.

Moreover, consuming a plant-based diet means you'll be consuming high amounts phytonutrients found only in plants; which, combined with the avoidance of the toxins found in meat, dairy, and eggs, have been shown to decrease the risk of cancer significantly. **There have actually been many cases of people having cancer, going vegan or vegetarian, and then curing themselves as a result. Rob Mooberry is one of those people.**

Rob had stage 4 colorectal cancer, and after chemotherapy, radiation, and invasive surgeries didn't work, doctors gave him only a few weeks to live. This didn't stop him, though. He was determined to do whatever it took to beat his cancer and stay alive, and that's when he switched his diet and went *"hardcore raw, vegan, superfoods."*

**After only a few months** (and living passed his death prognosis of only a few weeks), **when he returned to the hospital for a follow-up scan, it showed his cancer had** *"shrunk in size by nearly 80%. Fast forward almost a year from that scan, and [his] scans showed almost no evidence of the disease."*

Today, Rob is over six years cancer-free and has since started his own cancer charity, the **Mu Casa Moo Foundation,** that he uses to share his story of beating cancer with plants. [37]

The same thing goes with diabetes and heart disease. **A plant-based diet is the** *only* **thing** *proven* **through comprehensive medical research and real-world examples to** *reverse the effects of and cure,* **both type 2 diabetes and heart disease.** [20]

Furthermore, a plant-based diet also helps with Inflammatory Bowel Syndrome (IBS) and ulcerative colitis, as it can keep you in remission by lowering inflammation within the body, which then significantly reduces the need for harmful medications. Dr. Garth Davis **(@drgarthdavis),** the author of ***Proteinaholic*** (which I've referenced numerous times throughout this section), is an excellent example of this, as he used to have terrible IBS when he used to eat meat. But now that he's vegan, his IBS is completely gone! [20]

**In total, a plant-based diet has been shown to reverse the effects of (or even cure):**

- Cancer
- Diabetes
- Heart Disease
- Hypertension
- Rheumatoid Arthritis
- Diverticulosis
- Gallstone Disease
- Gout
- Cataracts
- Mental Illness [20]

Not only that, **I can personally say that a plant-based diet makes you feel so much better!** Since going vegetarian myself in November 2017, and then fully vegan in August 2018, my energy levels have been through the roof!

**My body always feels incredible!** I recover so much faster after workouts (and I work out often and intensely). I never get sick; never feel run down or sluggish. I consume caffeine very minimally. And sometimes I only get four to five hours of sleep at night, yet I always feel so full of energy and life! I'm the healthiest I've ever been, and my numbers show.

- As of November 2018, my **total cholesterol** is only **137.**
- My **HDL** level, **the healthy cholesterol,** which you want more of and not less (and, quoting my doctor, *"most people have a hard time getting theirs above 40"*), is **62.**
- My **triglycerides,** which should be under 150, are only **61.**
- And my **LDL** level, **the unhealthy cholesterol,** which should be under 100–is also only **61.**

Unfortunately, the only number I have to compare for reference from when I ate meat is my cholesterol, which was 178 in 2014. But seeing how low it is now, I can confidently say that it's due to my change in diet (because that's the only thing that's changed since then), and I can only imagine how high my other numbers were back during my meat-eating time.

## Ethical

This one is simple. By not consuming animal protein, you're no longer contributing to the suffering and killing of billions of innocent sentient beings each year. **And morally and spiritually, that makes me feel** *even better* **than how my body does!**

## Environmental

**Each day,** a person who eats a vegan diet saves:
- 1,110 gallons of water
- 45 pounds of grain
- 30 square feet of forest
- 20 pounds of $CO_2$ emission
- At least one animal's life

**Each year,** a person who eats a vegan diet saves:
- 401,500 gallons of water
- 16,425 pounds of grain
- 10,950 square feet of forest
- 730 pounds of $CO_2$ emission
- At least 365 animal lives

**In total,** a person who follows a vegan diet produces 50% less $CO_2$ than a meat eater; and uses $1/11^{th}$ less oil, $1/13^{th}$ less water, and $1/18^{th}$ less land. [5]

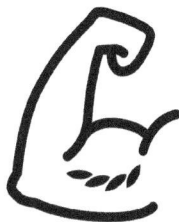

**2.6**

# Choices

Going vegan isn't something you need to do overnight, as I didn't either. Nor is it something you need to do at all. At the end of the day, what you choose to do is your choice, and I'll never tell you what you can or cannot do.

What I will ask of you, though, is to **think about how your actions affect others.** If not thinking in terms of your own health, **at least think about how eating meat and animal products affects the health of our planet and all of its living beings.**

The beauty of being human is that we can think cognitively about our choices, empathize with others, and then choose to act accordingly by doing what we would want to be done if we were that other creature.

Animal agriculture causes so much harm in so many ways. **Our planet needs *YOU*. The animals need *YOU*. You *CAN* make a difference! You just need to think bigger than yourself, and then start matching your actions with your beliefs.**

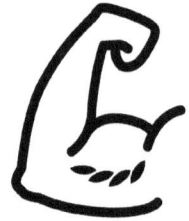

# My Story

I remember the last time I ate meat. It was Saturday night, November 11th, 2017. My mom, brother, and I were in Albany, NY to visit family and to see the last football game at Union College for the year.

That night, we went to The Cheesecake Factory for dinner and had a few different meat-based dishes. We shared buffalo chicken blasts for an appetizer, and spicy cashew chicken and chicken Bellagio pasta dishes for our main meal. And of course, we also had cheesecake for dessert. This type of heavy eating isn't uncommon for me when going to restaurants. I always eat relatively clean during the week and then occasionally on the weekends, I'll relax and have some larger not-so-healthy meals when I go out.

That summer, though, I had already been slowly cutting back my meat consumption, and then come the next morning following our meat-heavy dinner at Cheesecake, I woke up with my stomach feeling terrible.

**My brother and I then proceeded to watch *What the Health* in the hotel room, and after seeing everything that went on in the documentary, I vowed never to eat meat again.**

Fast forward to July 2018, the last time I knowingly ate any animal products also happened to be at The Cheesecake Factory on the 31st when my brother and I went to the one in Providence, RI for National

Cheesecake Day–which is funny because all of my closest family and friends know just how much I love The Cheesecake Factory (lol).

The last thing to go for me was the baked goods and sweets made with butter, eggs, and milk, which was hard because I have a big sweet tooth and I was also dealing with a period of post-show binging at the time (more on this in the "Meditation" chapter, page 227).

But my brother, who's basically my twin (although we're almost four years apart), made the transition to vegetarianism and then veganism with me. And during our time of being vegetarian, he'd always remind me of the evil of the egg and dairy industries.

> *"Yeah Bob, I know you like your cookies, but they're made with dairy and eggs; and just because those things aren't meat doesn't make it okay. You don't believe in the exploitation, suffering, or killing of animals; yet all animals of animal agriculture, including the chickens and cows of the egg and dairy industries, are exploited, suffer, and are ultimately killed for meat."*

And because of that constant reaffirmation from him, and me finally fully connecting with my *"why,"* I went vegan (and so did he), and we haven't looked back since!

**Thank you, bro.**

# Continued Education
# & Awareness

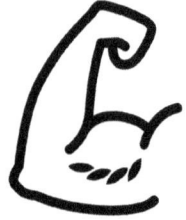

Some books, documentaries, and podcasts that have been very influential for me on my personal journey to and through veganism are listed below. I highly recommend reading, watching, and listening to them all, as they're very eye-opening and informative.

## Books

- *Finding Ultra,* Rich Roll
- *How Not to Die,* Dr. Michael Greger
- *Proteinaholic,* Dr. Garth Davis
- *The Blue Zones Solution,* Dan Buettner
- *The Cheese Trap,* Dr. Neal Barnard
- *The China Study,* Colin Campbell
- *The Starch Solution,* Dr. John McDougall

## Documentaries

- *What the Health*
- *Cowspiracy*
- *Dominion*
- *Earthlings*
- *Food Choices*
- *Food, Inc.*
- *Forks Over Knives*
- *Rotten*

- *The Game Changers*

## Podcasts
- *Generation V,* Nimai Delgado
- *Rich Roll Podcast,* Rich Roll
- *That Vegan Couple Podcast,* Natasha & Luca Padalini
- *The Disclosure Podcast,* Earthling Ed
- *The Exam Room,* The Physicians Committee
- *Plant Strength Radio,* Bobby Lynch ;)
  - *plantstrengthradio.com*

# Part 3

# Preparing to Win

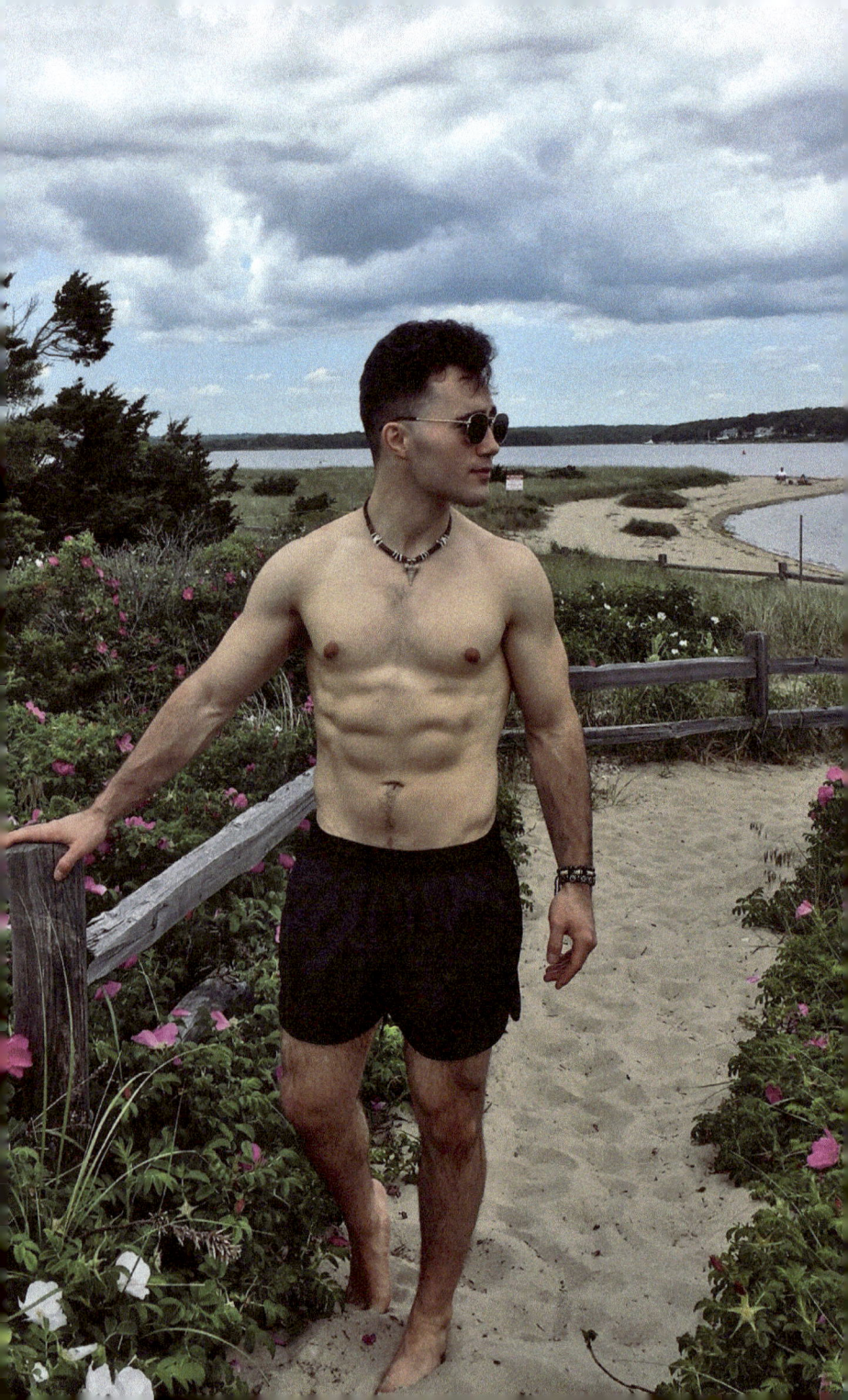

**3.1**

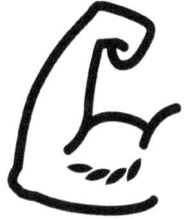

# Getting Organized

*"For every minute spent organizing, an hour is earned."*

– Benjamin Franklin

One of the biggest excuses that I hear for why someone *"can't exercise"* or *"eat healthily"* is because *"they don't have the time to."* But the truth is, **they DO!** The reason they *think* that they don't, however, is because **they haven't organized their schedule and made exercising and preparing healthy food a priority.**

**Every person has 168 hours each week to use how they please.** Yes, on average, most people will spend 40-50 of those hours working. But even if that number is 50, that still leaves you with 118 for yourself. Factor in another eight hours per night to sleep (56 total) and you're still left with 62.

To get and *stay* in great shape, ideally, three to four hours each week should be spent on purposeful exercise, and another three to four on food preparation. Meaning, *at most* **you need to spend eight hours each week focused on your health and fitness–less than *5%* of your weekly time.**

If you're telling me that you can't dedicate 5% of your time to your health (the *most important* thing in your life), then the only person you're fooling is yourself!

**To best organize your schedule,** first, you want to **know the hours you spend working,** which include your:
- Time at the office.
- Commute.
- Time to get ready in the morning.

For example, if you work the standard 9 am to 5 pm job, five days per week, but you have a 30-minute commute each way, and it takes you an hour to get ready every morning; then really, you're working 50 hours each week:
- 40 hours at the office
- 5 hours commuting
- 5 hours getting ready every morning

Once you know the exact hours you spend working, next, you'll want to **determine when your free-time hours are:**
- During the week (morning, afternoon, and night).
- On the weekends (and if you have any typical plans).

After that, I suggest you **buy a planner** (if you don't already own one). Personally, I have a big whiteboard calendar at home on the wall in my office, which gives me a visual overview of my schedule for the month and weeks ahead. I then sync all of what's on this calendar with my phone's calendar so that I can always see when I'm busy and when I'm free.

Once your basic schedule is in order, **schedule your health and fitness time.** When doing so, you must **treat each event like it's a business meeting that's *not* optional.** So, just as when your boss says you have a meeting on Tuesday at 1 pm, *"don't be late!"*–the same thing goes for your workouts and food preparation. **These are mandatory meetings with yourself for the benefit of your health, which, again, is *the most important thing in your life!***

If you're not healthy, then you won't be able to give your best self to anyone or anything (family, friends, career, hobbies; you name it). And because of that, you'll never reach your full potential or happiness.

**Organize your schedule and audit your time and you'll realize just how much more you actually have.**

# Shaping Your Environment

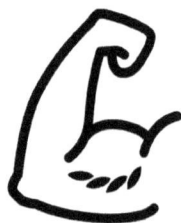

**John Berardi's First Law states:**

> *"If a food is in your house or possession, either you, someone you love, or someone you marginally tolerate, will eventually eat it."* [7]

This rings true for both healthy and unhealthy food. If you're always surrounded by processed snack foods, then processed snack foods are likely what you'll eat. But if you're always surrounded by whole foods like beans, fruit, whole grains, and vegetables, then whole foods are likely what you'll eat.

**Not only does the food in your environment affect your decision making, *who* is in it affects you, as well.** The saying, *"surround yourself with five successful people, and you'll be the sixth,"* is true.

If the people closest to you (especially the ones you live and work with) are supportive of your goals, then the likelihood of you staying motivated and achieving them will be high. But if these people aren't supportive and they don't keep you accountable or motivated, then they're only going to hold you back.

**So instead of letting your environment shape you, *shape it first* to set yourself up for success!**

**To shape your environment, start by assessing the following areas in your life:**
- Social Support
- Household
- Kitchen
- Office

Analyze how each currently is, ask questions to determine what's in your control, and then take action on what you can and let go of what you can't.

## Social Support

- Who in your life is the *most* helpful, encouraging, and supportive? How?
- Who in your life is the *least* helpful, encouraging, and supportive? How?
- Do any of these people live or work with you?

Unfortunately, you can't control who will support and who won't, but **you *can* control who you spend your time with.** Even if you live together. If the people you live with are helpful, encouraging, and supportive of your goals, then the more power to you! But if they're not, then have a talk with them.

Ask why they aren't supportive and explain the importance of your goals. If they respond positively and are willing to change their ways, then great! If not, then you'll have to limit your time with them. Do the same with your coworkers and close friends. **Keep your inner circle tight and full of *good vibes only!***

# Household

- Who does most of the grocery shopping in your household?
- Who does most of the cooking?
- Who decides on most of the menus and meal types?

Ideally, no matter who lives with you, you should have control over (or at least play an integral part in) the grocery shopping, cooking, and menu of your home.

If you live alone or if you live with roommates, but each of you does your own shopping, then this shouldn't be a problem.

But if you live with your spouse or parent(s) and they control the menu, then I also suggest having a chat with them. Explain your goals and how certain foods are more beneficial than others and that you'd like to incorporate more beneficial ones into the household diet, and less unhealthy ones. Hopefully, they'll respond positively and respect your wishes. If not, don't give up. **Stay positive and stay persistent!** Eventually, they're likely to come around. In the meantime, you might have to do some shopping and cooking for yourself.

# Kitchen

**The first kitchen assessment you'll want to make is of the food you already have.**

- What food and drinks are stored in your cupboards, freezer, fridge, and pantry?
    - Of these foods and drinks, list those that are nutrient-dense[4] and then those that are empty calories.[5]

---

[4] See the "Best Nutrient-Dense Foods" list, page 97.
[5] See the "Empty Calories" list, page 104.

- What nutrient-dense foods and drinks could you stock up on or add?
- What empty calories are you willing to part with or make more inconvenient to get to?

Remember, **the more you surround yourself with nutrient-dense food, the higher the chance you'll eat it and vice versa.**

If you already have plenty of nutrient-dense food at your disposable, then awesome! See if you need any more and add to your supply. If you don't, then the same thing applies. See what you need and then go get it!

If you have too many unhealthy and processed foods lying around, then be realistic and determine what you're willing to let go of now, and what you'd still like to keep for occasional enjoyment.

For the ones you're willing to let go of, toss them outside for the wildlife (if you live in an area where you can), or give them away to coworkers and friends. For the ones you keep, make them more inconvenient to get to. For example, **store your ice cream behind your frozen veggies in the freezer and your cookies behind your rice and beans in the pantry.**

**Keeping healthy nutritious options at your disposal and in the way of those that won't provide any nutrients will make you think twice about the food that you actually want (and need) the next time you have the urge to reach for unhealthy choices.** This doesn't mean though that you can never eat cookies, ice cream, or other empty calories—it's just about eating *less* of them.

**Next, assess the cleanliness and organization of your kitchen.**

On a scale of 1-10: 1 being *"chaos and filth,"* and 10 *"you-can-lick-the-floors clean";* how clean and organized is your kitchen?
- Are the counters and floor dirty?
- Is the sink full of dishes?
- Can you easily find your cooking equipment?
- Do you have all the cooking equipment you need?

Before you can begin to prepare food properly, you need to ensure your kitchen is properly cleaned and organized.
- Wipe down the counters
- Vacuum and sweep the floor
- Wash any dirty dishes
- Put away pans, pots, and utensils in a neat and orderly fashion

A dirty kitchen is uninspiring and unsanitary. But a clean kitchen is a happy kitchen, and a happy kitchen makes for a great (and sanitary) cooking experience. **You wouldn't want the cooks of your favorite restaurant preparing your food in a dirty kitchen, so why should you at home?**

Once your kitchen is cleaned, make sure that you have all the proper equipment needed to prepare food. Use the list below to crosscheck with what you already have and then add whatever you don't to this week's shopping list.

## Kitchen Equipment
- Baking Sheet(s)
- Blender/Food Processor *(High-Powered/High-Speed)*
  - *Ninja, NutriBullet, Vitamix*
- Chef Knife Set
- Colander/Strainer
- Cutting Board

- Food Scale
- Glass Bowls *(Small, Medium, Large)*
- Measuring Cups
- Measuring Spoons
- Non-Stick Aluminum Foil
- Non-Stick Frying/Sauté Pan(s)
- Ovenproof Casserole Dish
- Parchment Paper
- Pots *(Small, Medium, Large)*
- Rice Cooker/Instant Pot
- Spatula(s)
- Storage Containers
- Utensils *(Forks, Spoons, Knives)*
- Vegetable Peeler
- Wooden Spoon(s)

## Office

Lastly, assess your office environment because what you keep in your workspace will also make a big difference.

- Do you store food at your desk? If yes, what kind?
- Do you always have water at your desk? If yes, how often do you drink it?
- Are there food and drinks readily available to employees in the office? If yes, what kind?
- Do you bring your own lunch and snacks every day?

**Organize your office space just like you would your kitchen cabinets, freezer, fridge, and pantry.**

If you keep snacks at your desk, make sure they're healthy and nutritious (fruit, protein/granola bars, low-fat pretzels, fava beans, protein powder, etc.). But store them in a drawer so that they're out of sight and not a distraction.

**Always keep a water bottle on top your desk and in plain sight.** Dehydration, especially at the workplace, is common among many people. You get so caught up with what you're doing, you forget to take care of yourself. Staying hydrated will best keep you focused and productive.

**For the breakroom,** if there's food readily available, assess what's there. If it's mainly processed snack foods (chips, cookies, crackers, etc.), then talk with your boss or manager and see if more healthy options can be incorporated. Explain how this would be in the best interest of both you and your coworkers to have more nutritious food on hand. If he or she responds positively and changes are made, then great job! But if he or she doesn't (or if you'd prefer not to speak up), then the breakroom is an area you'll want to avoid.

**For lunch,** more often than not, you should bring your own. On the days you don't, apply the General Restaurant Tips from the "Flexible Dieting" section (page 201), and make choices that align with your goals.

Remember, this is *flexible dieting.* Your diet doesn't have to be perfect. But the more nutrient-dense food you keep around, the more you'll eat, the better you'll feel, and the easier it'll be to reach your goals.

**Shape your environment so that it's a *winning environment* and watch how quickly your success will come!**

# Part 4

# Food & Cooking

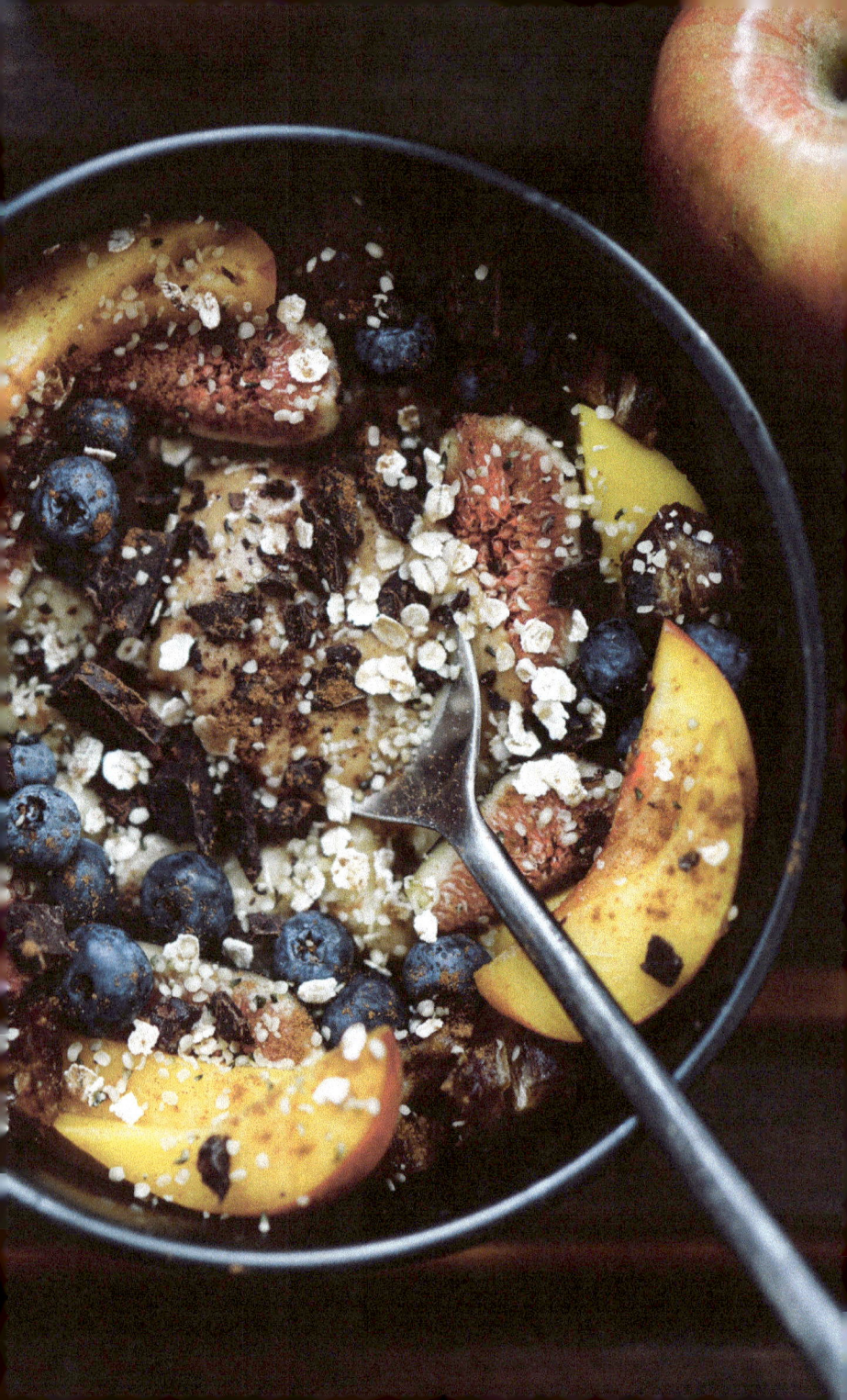

# Best Nutrient-Dense Foods (80%)

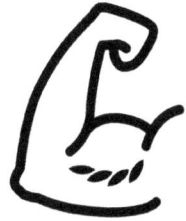

*Foods with a high nutrient content relative to their calories based on the micronutrients (vitamins, minerals, and phytochemicals) that they provide to your body.*

## Plant Protein

- Beans *(All sorts)*
- Broccoli
- Chickpea/Edamame/Lentil Pasta
- Chick'n Bites *(Made from Soy Flour)*
  - *Plant Strength (plantstrengthfoods.com)*
- Edamame (Soybeans)
- Mock Meat *(Vegan)*
  - *Beyond Meat, Boca, Field Roast, Gardein, Lightlife, Tofurky*
- Nutritional Yeast *(Also a great topping)*
- Peanut Butter Powder
- Peas
- Plant Milk/Soymilk
- Protein Bars *(Vegan)*
  - *Clif Builders, No Cow, Orgain, PROBAR, Sunwarrior*
- Protein Powder *(Vegan)*
  - *Garden of Life, Orgain, PEScience Vegan Select, Sunwarrior, Vega, Vivolife*
- Tempeh
- Textured Vegetable Protein (TVP) *(Made from Soy Flour)*

- Tofu
- Quinoa
- Seitan *(Made from Vital Wheat Gluten)*
  - *Upton's Naturals*

# Carbohydrates

- Amaranth
- Barley
- Buckwheat
- Bulgur
- Couscous
- Farro
- Kamut
- Legumes *(All sorts)*
- Millet
- Oatmeal
- Orzo
- Potatoes *(All sorts)*
- Rice *(All sorts)*
- Rice Cakes
- Sprouted Bread, Cereal, Grains, Granola
- Whole Grain Bread, Cereal, Granola, Pasta, Pita, Wraps
- Quinoa

## Fruit

- Apples
- Apricots
- Bananas
- Berries *(All sorts)*
- Cantaloupe
- Cherries

- Dates
- Dragon Fruit
- Grapes
- Grapefruit
- Guava
- Honeydew
- Kiwi
- Lemons
- Limes
- Mango
- Melon
- Oranges
- Papaya
- Peaches
- Pears
- Pineapple
- Plums
- Pomegranate
- Pumpkin
- Watermelon

## Vegetables

- Artichokes
- Asparagus
- Beets
- Bell Peppers
- Broccoli
- Brussels Sprouts
- Carrots
- Cauliflower
- Celery
- Corn

- Cucumbers
- Eggplant
- Garlic
- Green Beans
- Mushrooms
- Okra
- Onions
- Peas *(All sorts)*
- Radish
- Scallions
- Squash *(All sorts)*
- Sunchokes
- Tomatoes
- Water Chestnuts
- Zucchini

## Leafy Greens

- Arugula
- Baby Beet Greens
- Cabbage
- Chard
- Chinese Cabbage
- Collard Greens
- Curly Endive
- Dandelion
- Garden Cress
- Kale
- Mache
- Microgreens
- Mustard Greens
- Romaine
- Spinach

- Spring Mix
- Sprouts
- Tatsol
- Watercress

## Fat

- Almonds
- Avocado
- Brazil Nuts
- Cashews
- Chia Seeds
- Coconut
- Flaxseeds
- Hemp Seeds
- Hummus
- Macadamia
- Nut Butters *(All sorts)*
- Peanuts
- Pecans
- Pistachios
- Pumpkin Seeds
- Sunflower Seeds
- Tahini
- Vegan Cheese
  - *Daiya, Field Roast, Follow Your Heart*
- Walnuts

## Liquids

- Apple Cider Vinegar
- Almond Milk
- Banana Milk

- Cashew Milk
- Coconut Milk
- Coffee *(Black)*
- Iced Tea *(Unsweetened)*
- Kombucha
- Low-Calorie Sport Drinks
- Macadamia Nut Milk
- Oat Milk
- Plant Milk
- Protein Shakes *(See Protein Powder under Plant Protein)*
- Soymilk
- Tea
- Vegetable Broth
- **WATER**

## Low-Calorie Condiments, Sauces & Toppings

*50 Calories or Less per Two-Tablespoon Serving*

- Coconut Aminos
- Green/Red-Chile Sauce
- Hot Sauce
- Ketchup
- Liquid Aminos
- Low-Calorie BBQ Sauce
- Low-Calorie/Fat-Free Dressings
- Low-Calorie Syrup
- Low-Sodium Soy Sauce
- Mustard
- Pepper Sauce
- Relish
- Salsa
- Sriracha

- Tomato Sauce
- Tzatziki Sauce
- Vinegar
- Worcestershire Sauce

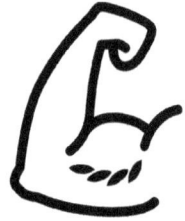

# Empty Calories (20%)

*Foods with low-nutritional value that are calorically dense; typically processed; and either very high in fat, preservatives, sodium, sugar, or all four.*

***Avoid the consumption of meat and animal products.***

- Alfredo Sauce
- Bagels
- Baked Goods
- Barbeque Sauce
- Beer
- Bread Sticks
- Brownies
- Butter
- Cake
- Calzones
- Candy
- Canned Meat
- Canola Oil
- Cereal
- Chinese Food
- Cheesecake
- Cinnamon Buns
- Cookies

- Coolattas
- Corn Oil
- Corn Syrup
- Crackers
- Creamy Dressings/Sauces
- Dairy Milk
- Deli Meat
- Donuts
- Fast Food
  - *McDonald's, KFC, Subway, Taco Bell, etc.*
- Fatty Beef *(Less than 90% lean)*
- French Fries
- French Toast
- Fried Food *(All sorts)*
- Frozen Yogurt
- Fruit Juice
- Grinders, Subs
- Gummies
- Honey
- Hot Pockets
- Hydrogenated Oils
- Ice Cream
- Jam, Jelly
- Juice Cocktails
- Margaritas
- Mayonnaise
- Milk Shakes
- Muffins
- Oil *(All sorts)*
- Onion Rings
- Pancakes
- Pesto

- Pie
- Pizza Dough
- Popcorn *(Buttered)*
- Pop Tarts
- Potato Chips
- Pretzels
- Processed Meat *(Sausage, Hot Dogs, etc.)*
- Refined Sugar
- Sugar-Coated Nuts
- Sweetened Beverages *(Tea, Juice, etc.)*
- Sweetened Nut Butters
- Sweetened Cottage Cheese
- Sweetened Yogurt
- Syrup *(All sorts)*
- Waffles
- White Bread
- White Flour
- White Pasta
- Wine

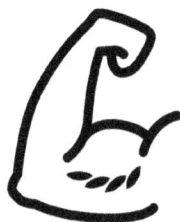

# Recipes

In this chapter, you'll find the recipes for how to cook almost every food from the "Best Nutrient-Dense Foods" list (page 97).

## Protein

### Beans

**Canned**

- Empty the can into a strainer and rinse the beans under cold water. Transfer the beans to a glass dish and add 3-4 ounces of water. Cook covered for 10-15 seconds per ounce depending on the wattage of your microwave (the higher the wattage, the less time necessary).
  - Thus, if you're cooking a 15-ounce can of beans, you'd cook them for 3-4 minutes.
- Once finished, drain the beans in a strainer and thoroughly rinse them again under cold water.

**Dried**

- **Sort:** Spread the dried beans on a baking sheet and sort through them to pick out any shriveled or broken beans, stones, or debris.
- **Cook:** Once sorted, place the beans in a large pot and cover with 2-3 inches of cold water above the top of the beans. Cover and bring to a boil on the stove. Once boiling, uncover the pot, reduce the heat to a simmer and cook until tender (about 60-90

minutes depending on the type of bean). Add water as necessary to keep the beans submerged. Add salt to taste (if desired).

## Lentils & Peas
**Canned**
- Same method as beans.

**Dried**
- **Sort:** Same method as beans.
- **Cook:** Pour 2-3 cups of cold water into a large pot for every 1 cup dried lentils/peas to be cooked. Bring the water to a boil and then add the lentils/peas. Once the water returns to a boil after the lentils/peas are added, reduce the heat to a simmer and cook partially covered until tender (about 30-45 minutes). Add salt to taste (if desired).

## Mock Meat (Vegan)
- Follow the cooking instructions on the bag, however, using water in place of oil when called for.

## Tempeh
**Prep**
- Slice your tempeh into strips or dice it into cubes. Marinate/season as desired. For a deeper flavor, place the coated tempeh in a container in the fridge and marinate overnight, or for at least 2-3 hours before cooking.

**Bake**
- While prepping, pre-heat your oven to 350°F. Place your tempeh on a non-stick baking sheet and then bake it in the oven at 350°F for 15-20 minutes.

**Grill**

- While prepping, heat your grill to medium heat. Place your tempeh on the grill and cook until it's browned but not burned (about 3-5 minutes). Flip, and then cook again until the reverse side is also browned but not burned (another 3-5 minutes, 6-10 minutes total).

**Sauté**

- While prepping, heat a skillet on the stove over medium heat. Place the tempeh in the skillet and then add water, soy sauce, or coconut/liquid aminos (avoid oil due to unnecessary calories). Cook until it's browned but not burned (about 3-5 minutes). Flip, and then cook again until the reverse side is also browned but not burned (another 3-5 minutes, 6-10 minutes total). Add additional water as needed to prevent the tempeh from sticking.

## Textured Vegetable Protein (TVP)

**Rehydrate**

- Combine 100 grams of TVP and 200 milliliters water, vegetable broth, or plant/nut milk (2:1, liquid:TVP ratio) to a large microwavable-safe dish. Cover and cook in the microwave on high for 3-4 minutes per 100 grams of TVP.
  - If rehydrating 200 grams, cook for 6-8 minutes; if 300 grams, cook for 9-12 minutes; etc.
- Mix the rehydrated TVP into any meal or recipe of choice as you would with meat.

## Tofu (Extra Firm)

**Prep**

- Open your tofu package and pour the tofu and water into a colander or strainer in the sink to drain the water. If the tofu came formed as a block, transfer it to a cutting board after the water is drained and slice it into strips or dice it into cubes. Marinate/season as desired.

**Crispy**

- While prepping the tofu, heat an oven-safe metal or cast-iron skillet on the stove over medium-low heat, and pre-heat your oven to 375°F.
- Once the burner is hot, add the tofu to the skillet. Add water, soy sauce, or coconut/liquid aminos (avoid oil due to unnecessary calories) and then sauté uncovered, stirring and flipping occasionally to cook the tofu on all sides. Add additional seasonings (as desired). Continue cooking until all the liquid in the pan has evaporated (about 8-10 minutes).
- Transfer the skillet to the oven and bake at 375°F until the tofu is firm to the touch and has begun to dry out and crisp up (about 15 minutes).

**Bake**

- While prepping, pre-heat your oven to 375°F. After prepping, place the tofu on a non-stick baking sheet and bake at 375°F for 20 minutes.

**Scramble**

- While prepping, heat a skillet on the stove over medium-low heat. Place the tofu in a bowl and crumble it with a fork until it reaches scrambled-egg consistency.
- Once the burner is hot, dump the tofu into the skillet and sauté it using the same method as Crispy minus baking it in the oven.

**Sauté**

- Same method as Crispy minus baking it in the oven.

# Carbs

## Amaranth

- Combine 0.5 cups of dry amaranth with 1.5 cups of water or vegetable broth in a large pot and stir. Cover and bring to a boil on the stove.
- Once boiling, reduce the heat to a simmer and cook partially covered, stirring occasionally for 15-20 minutes until all the liquid is absorbed. Add seasoning (if desired) and stir 1-2 minutes before finished cooking, just before the liquid fully absorbs. Pour the cooked amaranth into a large bowl and fluff with a fork before serving.

## Barley

**Hulled** (Bran layer still intact)

- Combine 1 cup barley with 2.5 cups of water or vegetable broth in a large pot. Cover and bring to a boil on the stove.
- Reduce the heat to a simmer and cook partially covered, stirring occasionally until tender (about 40-50 minutes), and most of the liquid has absorbed. Add seasoning (if desired) and stir 3-5 minutes before finished cooking, just before the liquid fully absorbs. Pour the cooked barley into a large bowl and fluff with a fork before serving.

**Pearled** (Bran layer removed)

- Combine 1 cup barley with 1.75 cups water or vegetable broth in a large pot. Cover and bring to a boil on the stove.
- Once boiling, reduce the heat to a simmer and cook partially covered, stirring occasionally until tender (about 10-15 minutes). Pour cooked Barley into a large bowl and fluff with a fork before serving.

## Bulgur

- Combine 1 cup bulgur with 1.5 cups water or vegetable broth in a large pot and stir. Cover and bring to a boil on the stove.
- Once boiling, reduce the heat to a simmer and cook partially covered, stirring occasionally until tender (about 10-15 minutes) and most of the liquid is absorbed. Add seasoning (if desired) and stir 1-2 minutes before finished cooking, just before the liquid fully absorbs. Drain the cooked bulgur in a colander, pour it into a large bowl, and then fluff with a fork before serving.

## Couscous

- Combine 1 cup dry couscous with 1 cup water or vegetable broth in a large pot and stir. Cover and bring to a boil on the stove.
- Once boiling, remove the pot from the heat and steam for 5-7 minutes. Drain the cooked couscous in a colander, pour it into a large bowl, add seasoning (if desired), and then fluff with a fork before serving.

## Farro

- Combine 1 cup dry farro with 3 cups water or vegetable broth in a large pot and stir. Cover and bring to a boil on the stove.
- Once boiling, reduce the heat to a simmer and cook uncovered, stirring occasionally until tender (about 15-20 minutes). Drain the cooked farro in a colander, pour it into a large bowl, add seasoning (if desired), and then stir before serving.

## Kamut

- Combine 1 cup dry kamut with 3 cups water or vegetable broth in a large pot and stir. Cover and bring to a boil on the stove.

- Once boiling, reduce the heat to a simmer and cook covered, stirring occasionally until tender (about 60 minutes). Drain the cooked kamut in a colander, pour it into a large bowl, add seasoning (if desired), and then stir before serving.

## Millet

- Combine 1 cup dry millet with 2.5 cups water or vegetable broth in a large pot and stir. Cover and bring to a boil on the stove.
- Once boiling, reduce the heat to simmer and cook covered, stirring occasionally until tender (about 20-25 minutes). Drain the cooked millet in a colander, pour it into a large bowl, add seasoning (if desired), and then stir before serving.

## Oatmeal

### Instant Quick Oats

- Combine 0.5 cups (40 grams) oats with 0.75 cups water (180 milliliters) or 0.5 cups plant/nut milk (120 milliliters) in a medium microwavable-safe bowl. Cover and microwave on high for 90 seconds. Remove the cooked oats from the microwave, stir, and then let stand for 2 minutes.

### Steel-Cut Oats

- Combine 0.25 cups steel-cut oats with 1 cup water (240 milliliters) or 0.75 cups (180 milliliters) plant/nut milk in a medium saucepan, stir, and bring to a boil on the stove.
- Once boiling, reduce the heat to a simmer and cook uncovered, stirring occasionally for 25-30 minutes, or until the oats are of your desired texture.

## Orzo

- Pour 3 quarts (12 cups) water into a large pot and stir in 1 tablespoon of sea salt (if desired). Cover and bring to a boil on the stove.
- Add 1 cup dry orzo and boil until firm and chewy (about 10 minutes), stirring occasionally to prevent sticking. Drain the cooked orzo in a colander when finished.

## Pasta

- Pour 5 quarts (20 cups) of water into a large pot and stir in 4 tablespoons of sea salt (if desired). Cover and bring to a boil on the stove.
- Add your desired amount of pasta to the water, stir gently, and then let the water return to a boil. Continue boiling uncovered, stirring occasionally for 8-10 minutes. Remove the cooked pasta from the heat and drain in a colander.

## Potatoes
**Oven**

- Pre-heat your over to 400°F. Thoroughly wash potatoes under cold running water, skin (if desired), and slice/dice potatoes as desired. If cooking the potatoes whole, evenly poke holes on all sides with a fork or knife before cooking.
- Place potatoes on a non-stick baking sheet, add seasoning (if desired), and bake at 400°F for 30-40 minutes.

**Microwave**

- Thoroughly wash your potatoes under cold running water and skin (if desired). Evenly poke holes on all sides with a fork or knife before cooking.
- Place the potatoes on a plate, cover, and cook on high for 5-15 minutes depending on the amount/size of the potatoes.

o    Larger/more potatoes equals more time and vice versa.

## Rice
- Combine 1 cup rice with 2.5 cups water or vegetable broth in a large pot and stir. Cover and bring to a boil on the stove.
- Once boiling, reduce the heat to a simmer and cook covered, stirring occasionally until tender (about 40-50 minutes). Drain the cooked rice in a colander, pour it into a large bowl, add seasoning (if desired), and then fluff with a fork before serving.

## Quinoa
- Combine 1 cup dry quinoa with 2 cups water or vegetable broth in a large pot and stir. Cover and bring to a boil on the stove.
- Once boiling, reduce the heat to a simmer and cook partially covered, stirring occasionally for 15-20 minutes until the liquid is absorbed. Add seasoning (if desired) and stir 1-2 minutes before finished cooking, just before the liquid fully absorbs. Pour the cooked quinoa into a large bowl and then fluff with a fork before serving.

# Vegetables
## Corn
### On the Cob
- Remove the husks and silk from the corn. Fill a large pot with cold water until 75% full and bring the water to a boil on the stove. Stir in 2 tablespoons sea salt, 2 tablespoons sugar, and 1 tablespoon lemon juice (if desired), dissolving the salt and sugar.
- Gently place the ears of corn into the boiling water and cover the pot. Turn off the heat and let the corn cook in the hot water

until tender (about 10 minutes). Remove the cooked corn with tongs and season (if desired).

**Kernels from Frozen**

- Same method as for frozen vegetables.

## Frozen

**Microwave**

*This method can be applied to all vegetables.*

- Pour frozen vegetables into a large microwavable-safe dish. Add 2 ounces of water for every 8 ounces of vegetables. Cover and cook on high for 3-4 minutes.
  - For example, for 16 ounces of vegetables, you'd cook them for 6-8 minutes.
- Remove the cooked vegetables from the microwave, drain them in a colander, and then thoroughly rinse under cold running water.

**4.4**

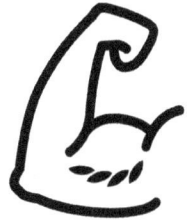

# Grocery Shopping

Building a well-balanced diet starts with your groceries, and healthy shopping starts before you're at the store. It starts with your list. Below are my steps to mastering healthy grocery shopping.

## 1. Make a List

Using the "Best-Nutrient Dense Foods" list (page 97), start by creating your own personalized "Favorite Healthy Foods" list, which includes all of your favorite nutrient-dense foods categorized by their main macronutrient.

Next, create a personal "Healthy Foods to Try" list of nutrient-dense foods that you've never had before but would be interested in trying. Again, categorize them by their main macronutrient for ease of reading.

Save these lists in your phone Notes so that you can refer to them wherever you are.

Before going to the store each week, decide on what you'd like to eat by choosing a few of your favorite nutrient-dense foods from each category, and at least one new food to try. Switch up your weekly choices to keep a variety, which prevents boredom and helps with maintaining a well-balanced diet.

## 2. Produce First

When you go to the store, always start in the produce section. Hopefully, the list of your favorite foods is full of a variety of colorful fruit and vegetables, and your cart should be too. The color reflects the respective micronutrient content, so buying a variety ensures you'll obtain all the necessary vitamins, minerals, and phytochemicals that you need.

If your budget allows, **I recommend buying organic produce because it contains far fewer (or zero) pesticides and is usually more flavorful.** However, it does come at a higher cost and so if you're looking to save money, go with regular produce instead, just make sure to wash it thoroughly before eating.

To know whether your produce is conventionally grown, organic, or genetically modified, look at the PLU code on its label.
- **Conventionally grown** produce will have a four-digit code, usually beginning in a 3 or 4 like, "3129" or "4030."
- **Organic** produce is typically grouped together and clearly labeled as *"organic"* in the store, but it'll also have a five-digit code beginning with a 9 on its label like, "95864."
- **Genetically modified** produce will also have a five-digit code, but starting with an 8 like, "85864."

When buying fresh produce, it's always best to buy when it's in season, as in-season produce is not only more flavorful but also cheaper. Check out the **USDA Seasonal Produce Guide** to find the best time of year to buy your favorite fruit and veggies.

## 3. Read Ingredients & Nutrition Facts

After the produce, make your way through the subsequent isles. The ones directly following the produce section are usually the natural and organic isles that contain your natural and organic shelf foods (beans, bread, cereal, grains, pasta, etc.).

Again, although buying organic is your best bet because of the non-existent added chemicals, fillers, and preservatives, organic food is more expensive, and so if spending the extra money isn't something you'd like to do, that's perfectly okay.

**Be attentive to the ingredients list and stick to real foods for which you know what the ingredients are.** If what you're reading looks like an excerpt from a chemistry textbook, then it's probably full of additives and preservatives and isn't the best for you.

### Ingredients to Avoid

On the next page is a table of unhealthy and potentially harmful ingredients in processed food that you should aim to avoid, or at least minimize, in your diet due to their adverse effects on the body. At first glance, this list might seem overwhelming and you may be wondering how you'll remember it all, but don't stress because you don't need to.

When reading labels, again, **stick to foods with ingredients that you know. The smaller the ingredient list, the closer the food is to its natural state.** If a foreign ingredient appears when reading a label, simply crosscheck it with this list, or pull out your phone and do a quick google search to learn more about it. If it checks off as okay, then continue with your purchase. If it doesn't, then you might want to reconsider.

## Ingredients to Avoid

| | |
|---|---|
| Acesulfame Potassium | Guar Gum |
| Artificial/Natural Flavors | High Fructose Corn Syrup |
| Aspartame | Locust Bean Gum |
| Autolyzed Yeast Extract | Maltodextrin |
| Azodicarbonamide | Methylparaben |
| BHA | Monoglycerides and Diglycerides |
| BHT | Monosodium Glutamate |
| Bleached Flour | Neotame |
| Blue #1 | Partially Hydrogenated Oils |
| Calcium Peroxide/Propionate | Potassium Benzoate |
| Canola Oil | Propyl Gallate |
| Caramel Color | Propylparaben |
| Carrageenan | Red #3, Red #40 |
| Cellulose | Sodium Benzoate/Nitrate/Nitrite/Phosphate |
| Citric Acid | Soybean Oil |
| Corn Oil/Syrup | Soy Protein Isolate |
| Cottonseed Oil | Sucralose |
| DATEM | Synthetic Vitamins |
| Dextrose | TBHQ |
| Dimethylpolysiloxane | Titanium Dioxide |
| Enriched Flour | Vanillin |
| Fructose Syrup | Yeast Extract |
| Gellan Gum | Yellow #5, Yellow #6 |

[24]

## Non-Vegan Ingredients

For my fellow vegans, although you may think that the best vegan food-check is by looking at the allergen statement and so long as it doesn't contain meat, eggs, or dairy of any sort (milk, butter, cheese, etc.), then that food is vegan. Unfortunately, it's not that simple.

There are many additives derived from animals in processed foods that would otherwise appear vegan-friendly but are actually not because of them. Below are seven non-vegan ingredients to avoid that you may not have realized weren't vegan beforehand. [29] And don't worry, I was just as shocked when I learned of all of these too.

**Beeswax and Honey**
If you're sticking to the true definition of veganism, which seeks to exclude the exploitation of all living beings, then beeswax and honey are two things you'll want to avoid. Both are produced by bees:
- Beeswax for the building of their honeycombs.
- Honey for their food in the winter.

Beeswax is commonly used in lip balms and lotions, and honey is added as a sweetener in a variety of food or sold on its own.

**Casein**
Casein is derived from milk and is sometimes included in non-dairy foods, such as soy cheese or coffee creamers, as well as protein powder. You'll find it listed in ingredients as casein, calcium caseinate, or sodium caseinate.

**Confectioner's Glaze**
Mostly found on glossy candies like Candy Corn, Junior Mints, Red Hots, Lemonhead, and Boston Baked Beans, confectioner's glaze is made using the secretions from lac bugs (beetles). It'll appear in ingredients as confectioner's glaze, natural glaze, pure food glaze, resinous glaze, or shellac.

*Sounds delicious!*

### Gelatin

Gelatin is a colorless odorless gelling agent found in candy and other processed foods, the most well-known being Jell-O. It's derived from the skin, bones, and connective tissues of cattle, chicken, pigs, and fish.

*Tasty!*

### Isinglass

Used when making wine and brewing beer, isinglass is a clarifying agent derived from fish bladders.

*Yum!*

If you're unsure whether your drink is vegan-friendly, search the database at **barnivore.com** to see if it is or not, which contains over 42,000 beer, wine, and liquor products.

### L. Cysteine

L. Cysteine is a dough conditioner found in some pre-packaged baked goods and bread that's often sourced from feathers or human hair.

*Give me seconds!*

### Whey

Also derived from dairy as a byproduct of cheese making, whey is best known as the main ingredient in many protein powders but is also commonly found in bread and candies.

## Nutrition Facts

Ideally, the foods you buy should be either:
- High in fiber
- High in protein

- Full of vitamins and minerals
- Low in saturated and trans-fat
- Relatively low in calories per serving (caloric density)
- All of the above

## 4. Capitalize on Discounts & Sales

Typically, the discounts and sales at grocery stores are for cardholders only, which is why becoming a rewards member of your most-frequented supermarket is a game-changer when it comes to saving money.

On average, **I save between $10-15/week when I shop at my local Stop n' Shop just from being a rewards member and capitalizing on the weekly sales they're running, which totals between $500-800 in savings per year!** Often, I don't actually decide on what I want to eat that week until I'm already at the store because a lot of what I buy is determined by what's on sale.

Using coupons also helps increase my savings, as I'll either get them via flyers in the mail, or they'll be printed at the register at checkout for use during my next visit. Although, I do tend to forget my coupons at home a lot and so I now try keeping them in my car to always have them with me. Emphasis on *"try"* (lol).

## 5. Buy in Bulk

Another great way to save money is through purchasing large quantities of food at once (aka **bulk buying**).

**The best foods to buy in bulk are:**
- Beans
- Frozen Vegetables
- Grains

- Legumes
- Nutritional Yeast
- Nuts
- Oatmeal
- Pasta
- Protein Powder
- Rice
- TVP
- Vital Wheat Gluten

Nutritional yeast, TVP, and vital wheat gluten are three lean protein sources that I always buy in bulk because they last a while and are much cheaper than when buying them in smaller packages.

## 6.  Buy Frozen & Pre-Cut

In addition to buying dry foods in bulk, I also buy big bags of frozen fruit and vegetables. The fruit I use in my smoothies is almost always frozen and the same with the veggies in all of my meal preps.

**Frozen fruit and vegetables are great because they're both convenient and have more nutrients, as they're picked when ripe and then immediately frozen before being packaged for retail, which locks in the nutrients. As opposed to fresh fruit and veggies, which are picked *before* they're ripe and then shipped while exposed to air, which decreases their nutrient content.**

I also like to buy fresh pre-cut fruit and vegetables if I'm on-the-go, or when I'm having a busy week. It's more expensive to do this, however, but I'm willing to trade a couple extra dollars for convenience as necessary, if it means getting the nutrients that I need.

## 7. Frequent Co-ops & Farmers' Markets

When and where available, I highly recommend frequenting co-ops and farmers' markets. They always have the freshest produce that's locally grown, along with some of the best organic and vegan treats (for my fellow sweet connoisseurs). Not only will you find fresh excellent tasting food, but you'll also support your local community—*a win-win!*

## 8. Don't Shop Hungry

Last, but certainly not least, ***don't shop while hungry!*** It's never a good idea. *Trust me!* It leads to many impulsive decisions (typically unhealthy and processed ones), which are definitely what you want to avoid.

Have a snack or meal before you go, bring a large water bottle with you, apply the seven steps above, and *shop 'til you drop!* Under the weight of all of your fruit and vegetables, that is. ;)

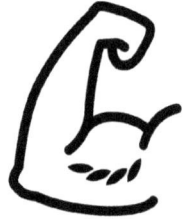

# Batch Cooking

*"By failing to prepare, you are preparing to fail."*

– Benjamin Franklin

**No matter your goals, whether they're health-, work-, or life-related, *preparation is key*.** If your goal is to get (and stay) in shape, then cooking food ahead of time is one of the best ways to ensure that you not only reach your goals but *maintain your results!*

We've all had those moments where, when it comes time to eat, you have no idea what to do because you have no food readily available–no healthy, nutrient-dense food that is. But those potato chips are sitting in the cabinet, calling your name. And so, what do you do?

*You answer their call.*

Trust me, I've been there many times myself. So, how do I make sure that I always have nutritious food on hand and ready for me to eat? *I batch cook!*

## Steps to Batch Cooking

### 1. Determine Quantity of Meals

If you're like me and it's convenient for you to make breakfast and dinner daily, then cooking for only one or two meals per day will suffice. However, if your schedule is busy, or if you prefer not having to cook every day, then cooking enough for two or more meals will be beneficial.

Determine how many meals per day you'll want to cook for and then multiply that quantity by the number of days you'll want that food to last (one meal per day times five days; two meals per day times six; etc.).

## 2. Determine Amount of Food per Meal

Figure out a rough average of how much you want to eat per meal (the amount of protein, carbs, veggies, and fat in ounces or grams), then multiply those serving sizes by your number of meals.

For example, for lunch, I typically eat six to eight ounces of protein, eight to 12 ounces of carbs, six to eight ounces of veggies, and one to two ounces of fat. Thus, when I go shopping, I multiply each of those serving sizes by seven and then buy the corresponding amount of each macronutrient. This means that I buy a combined total of:

- 42-56 ounces of protein (seitan, tofu, tempeh, mock meat, etc.).
- 56-84 ounces of carbs (beans, couscous, potatoes, rice, quinoa, etc.)
- 42-56 ounces of veggies (asparagus, broccoli, Brussels sprouts, green beans, etc.).
- Seven to 14 ounces of fat (avocado, hummus, nuts, seeds, etc.).

## 3. Buy Food Storage Containers

For your food storage, you have two options:
   A.  Store your food in large containers and portion out your meals each day, re-using one small container. This is considered **batch cooking.**

B.  Pre-portion your food into individual meals and store them in many small containers based on the amount of food you cooked. This is considered **meal prepping.**[6]

Personally, I prefer **batch cooking** over **meal prepping,** as it reduces the number of containers I need, which makes the food easier to store in my fridge; but to each his own.

## 4.  Schedule Time to Cook

Block off two to three consecutive hours on one or two days of every week to cook your food. Typically, Sundays are the day for me, and I prepare all of my food for the week. Occasionally, I'll split my cooking over two days and cook some of my food on Sunday; then the rest on either Wednesday or Thursday. Again, to each his own. Over time, you'll figure out what works best for you.

## 5.  Cook the Foods that Take the Longest, First

Food cooked in the oven most always takes the longest. So, if I'm cooking Seitan that week (which takes 60 minutes), I always start by cooking that first.

## 6.  Prep & Cook at the Same Time

The goal is efficiency; so, once you start cooking one thing, start preparing for the next.

## 7.  Use Multiple Cooking Sources

Continuing on the notion of efficiency, using multiple cooking sources will allow you to cook many things at once. For example, you could be

---

[6] See "Meal Prepping," page 179.

baking seitan in the oven, while cooking tofu and boiling quinoa on the stove, and steaming vegetables in the microwave–all at the same time.

## 8.  Clean Up as You Go

As soon as you finish cooking or prepping something, clean up any remnants right away (food packages, pans, pots, etc.). This will not only leave you with more counter space to work with while you continue to cook; but it'll also expedite the process, as you won't be left with a big mess still to clean once finished.

# Sample Batch Cooking Plan

## Food

- Broccoli
- Brussels Sprouts
- Couscous
- Tofu
- Quinoa
- Seitan

## Order of Operations

1. Pre-heat your oven and start prepping your Seitan.
2. Place the prepped Seitan in the oven and bake for 60 minutes. Clean up any Seitan prep remnants.
3. Take out a pot to cook your quinoa and turn on a stovetop burner.
4. Fill the pot with the required amount of water to cook the quinoa, and then add the quinoa to the pot.
5. Bring the water and quinoa to a vigorous boil, and then reduce the heat and simmer for 12-15 minutes.
6. While your quinoa is cooking, turn on a second stovetop burner and take out a frying pan to steam your tofu.

7. Start cooking the tofu while your quinoa is simmering.
8. Remove your quinoa from the stove once it's finished cooking and put it away in a large storage container.
9. Remove your Seitan from the oven once it's finished cooking and put it away in a large storage container.
10. Remove your tofu from the stove once it's finished cooking and put it away in a large storage container.
11. Clean up the baking dish, frying pan, and pot from the Seitan, tofu, and quinoa.
12. Re-use your quinoa pot to cook your couscous.
13. Add water and the couscous to the pot and cook covered on the stove, stirring occasionally.
14. Start prepping your broccoli while your couscous is cooking. Steam the broccoli in the microwave for 15 minutes.
15. Prep your Brussels sprouts while the broccoli is cooking. Clean up any broccoli and Brussels sprout prep remnants.
16. Remove your broccoli from the microwave once it's finished cooking and steam your Brussels sprouts for 15 minutes.
17. Cool off the broccoli under cold, running water and put it away in a large storage container while your Brussels sprouts are cooking.
18. Remove your Brussels sprouts from the microwave once they're finished cooking and cool them off under cold, running water. Put them away in a large storage container.
19. Remove your couscous from the stove once it's finished cooking and put it away in a large storage container.
20. Clean up anything leftover.

In total, this batch cooking plan should take two to three hours to complete. If you've never batch cooked before, then the first few times might take a bit longer, as you get used to the flow. Over time though, you'll develop a system that works best for *you,* and you'll become faster and more efficient.

**Batch cooking is a valuable tool that will *only help* you reach your goals. Give it a go and see just how beneficial it can be!**

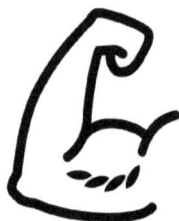

# Buddha Bowls

One of my favorite ways to create a meal is by mixing together a bunch of nutrient-dense foods and then topping them with a delicious dressing or sauce. I call these creations **Buddha Bowls.**

Buddha Bowls are great because they allow you to bring variety to your diet, which is one of the most common problems I see people struggle with—*a lack of variety*. Making Buddha Bowls is a fun way to get creative and mix things up, and I've outlined the exact blueprint below that I use to make my own.

## Buddha Bowl Blueprint

### 1.   Choose Your Base

Start by choosing one to two starchy carbs or whole grains as your base to the bowl (page 98). These will provide the bulk of your meal. My favorites are potatoes of all sorts (especially Japanese sweet potatoes), quinoa, corn, rice, and couscous. Beans and lentils may also serve as a base, as well as a protein.

If you're making a salad, choose some leafy greens as your base (page 100), and then add extra carbs on top if you'd like. My go-to leafy greens are baby spinach, kale, arugula, and spring mix.

## 2.  Add Protein

Next, add one to two lean protein sources like Seitan, tempeh, tofu, TVP, edamame, beans, lentils, or mock meat (page 97).

## 3.  Add Vegetables (and Fruit)

After your protein, add your vegetables (page 99). My favorite cooked veggies are broccoli, brussels sprouts, carrots, cauliflower, peas, and a mixed veggie blend. My favorite raw ones are beets, bell pepper, cucumber, mushrooms, onions, red cabbage, and tomato. Typically, I go with more cooked vegetables when making hot bowls and more raw ones when making salads.

Fruit is another great option to add sweetness to your bowl (page 98). My favorite raw fruits for bowls and salads are apples, bananas, blueberries, grapes, and strawberries; while my favorite dried ones are apples, bananas, craisins, and raisins.

## 4.  Add Fat

To ensure a healthy balance to your meal, round things out by adding some fats (page 101). My favorites are avocado, cashews, pistachios, shredded coconut, chia, flax, and hemp seeds. You may also obtain fats through your dressing or sauce; but be aware that most dressings are generally made with an oil base, and oil isn't the best for you.

## 5.  Season for Added Flavor

Before adding my dressing, I always sprinkle on some seasoning for extra flavor. My go-to seasonings are adobo, black pepper, chipotle powder, garlic powder, and nutritional yeast as they mix well with almost every dish.

### 6. Top with a Dressing or Sauce

Last, but certainly not least, it's time for the dressing! This is my favorite part; not only because it's the final step before sitting down to eat, but it's also the one that ultimately determines the overall flavor of the bowl. Use your favorite dressing, sauce, or topping or try something new (page 102). Pour it on, mix everything up, and delve into the wonders of your custom Buddha Bowl!

If you'd prefer to not go with a salad dressing, then go with a sauce or topping instead like BBQ, hot sauce, salsa, or whatever you'd like. This is your creation, and you can do with it anything you please!

Personally, I love adding coconut aminos to all of my bowls and salads, whether or not I'm adding another dressing or sauce, because they add *tremendous flavor!* Avoid the use of oils as they're highly processed, calorically dense, and provide little nutritional value relative to the number of calories.

## Buddha Bowl Samples

The following buddha bowls were all taken from my Instagram (**@bobbyphysique).**

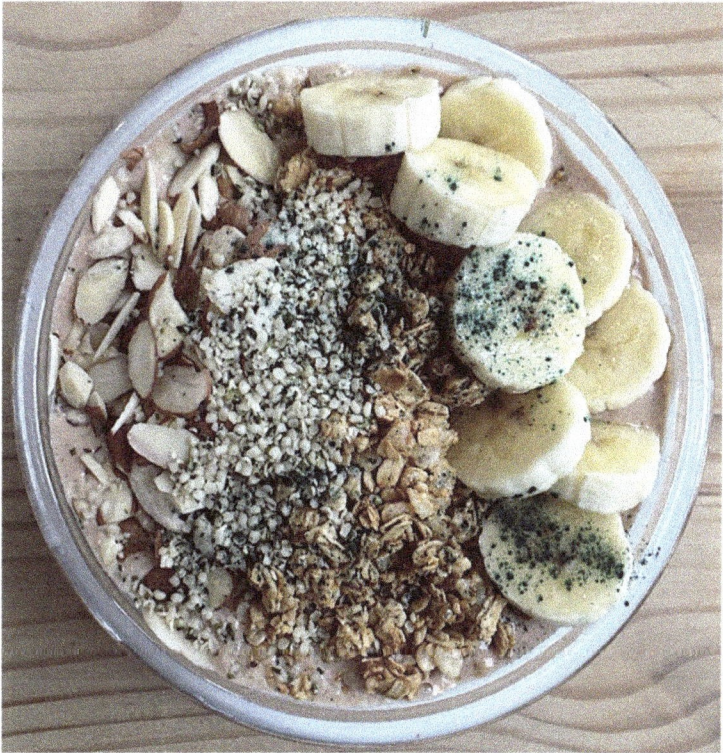

- **Base/Carbs:** Blended Pea Protein Powder, Peanut Butter, Banana, Medjool Date, Flaxseeds, Raw Cacao & pH 7.0 Filtered Water with Granola on Top
- **Protein:** Pea Protein Powder
- **Fruit:** Banana & Dates
- **Fat:** Flaxseeds, Hemp Seeds, Peanut Butter & Sliced Almonds
- **Seasoning:** Spirulina

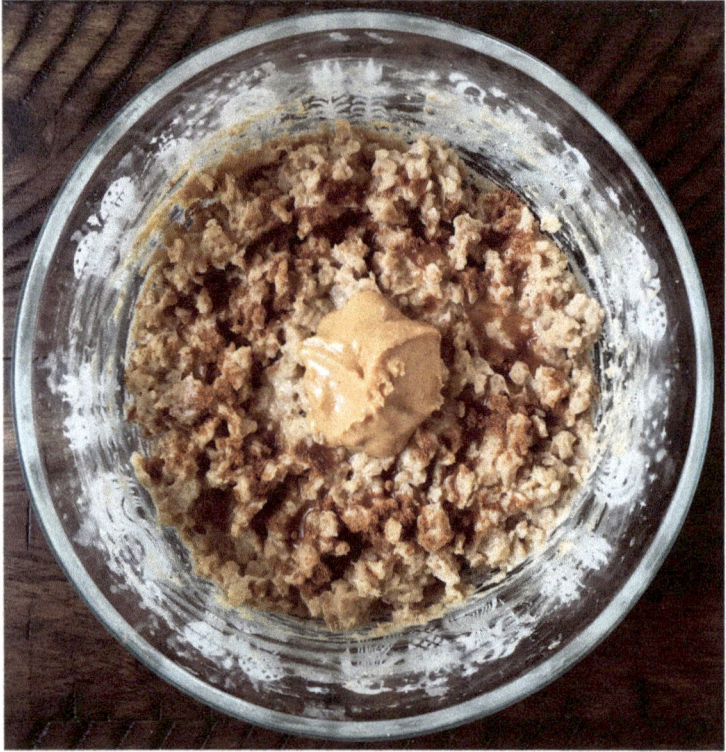

- **Base/Carbs:** Rolled Oats Heated in Unsweetened Vanilla Almond Milk
- **Protein:** PEScience Vegan Peanut Butter Delight Protein Powder
- **Fat:** Peanut Butter
- **Seasoning:** Ground Cinnamon

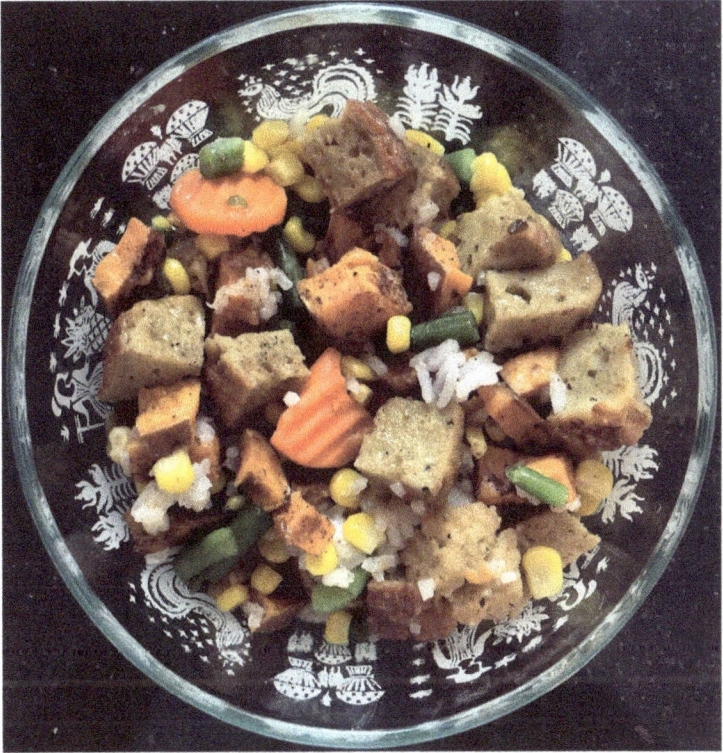

- **Base/Carbs:** White Rice
- **Protein:** Seitan
- **Veggies:** Carrots, Corn & Green Beans (Cooked from Frozen)
- **Fat:** Cashews & Pistachios
- **Seasoning:** Adobo & Garlic Powder
- **Dressing:** Sesame Ginger

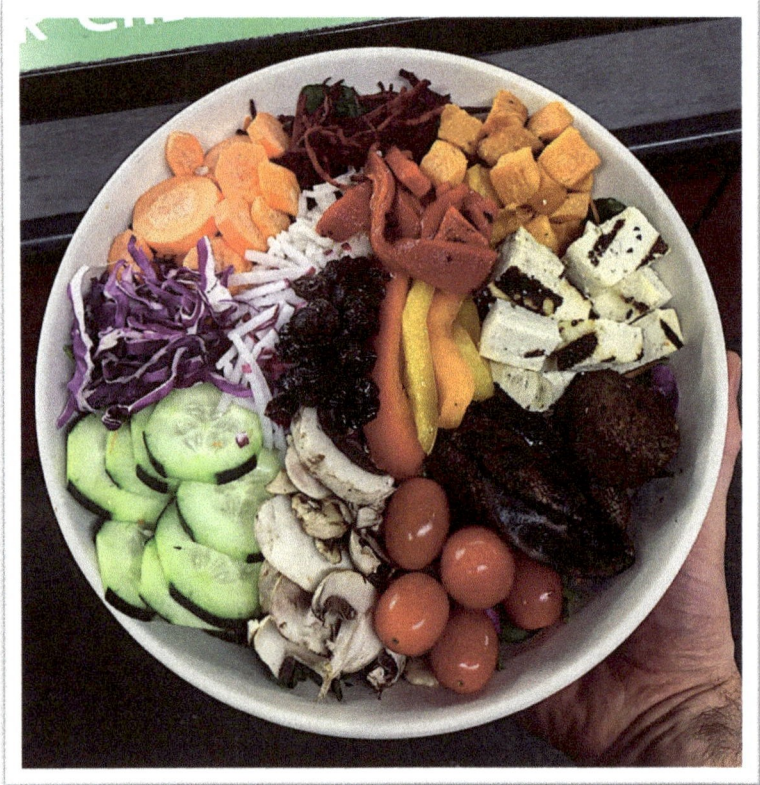

- **Base/Carbs:** Baby Spinach & Sweet Potatoes
- **Protein:** Grilled Tofu
- **Fruit & Veggies:** Beets, Bell Pepper, Carrots, Cherry Tomatoes, Cucumber, Portobello Mushrooms, Red Cabbage, Roasted Red Pepper, Radish, Raisins & White Mushrooms
- **Fat:** Falafel
- **Dressing:** Roasted Red Pepper

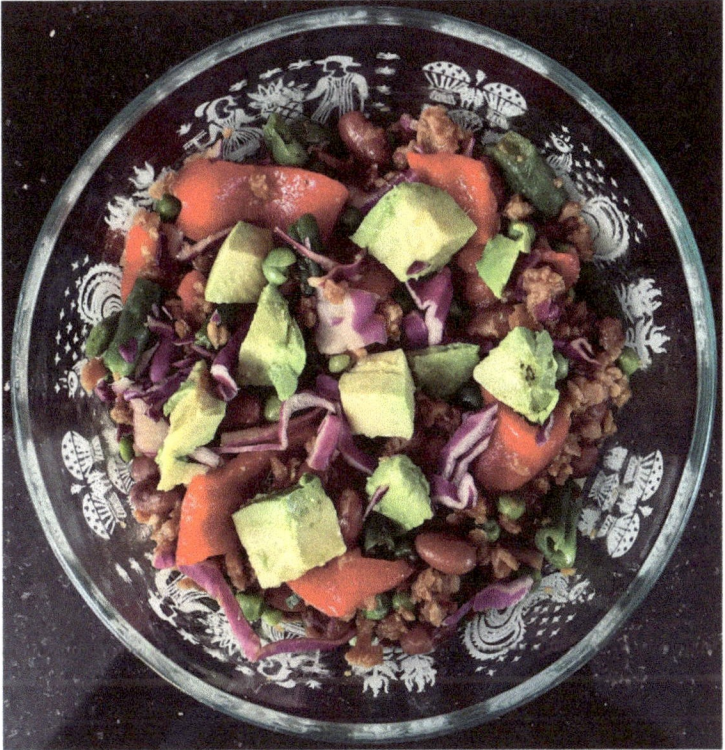

- **Base/Carbs:** Pink Beans
- **Protein:** Gardein Beefless Crumbles
- **Veggies:** Green Beans, Peas, Red Cabbage & Roasted Red Pepper
- **Fat:** Avocado
- **Seasoning:** Adobo & Garlic Powder
- **Dressing:** Citrus Ginger

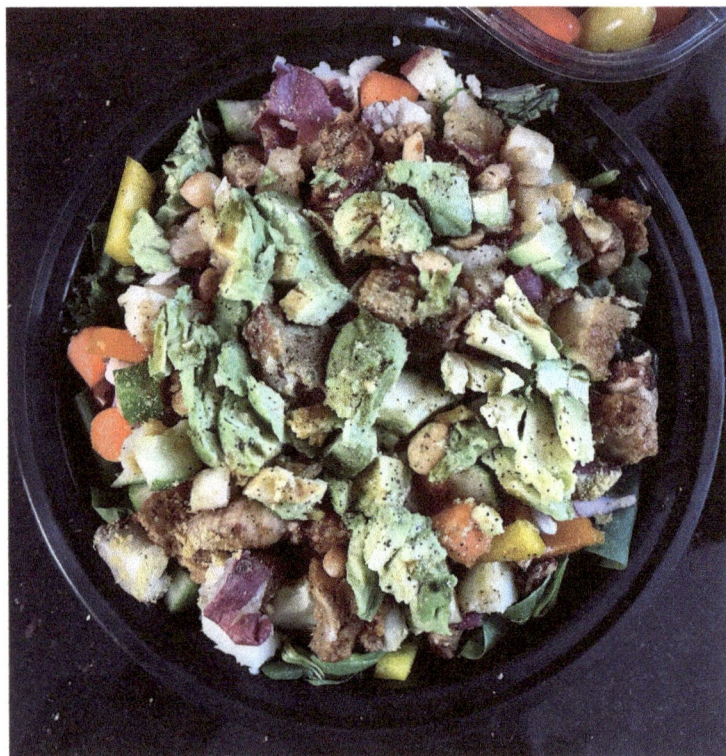

- **Base/Carbs:** Baby Spinach, Collard Greens, Kale & Red Potatoes
- **Protein:** Seitan
- **Veggies:** Bell Pepper, Carrots, Cucumber, Red Cabbage & Vidalia Onion
- **Fat:** Avocado & Mixed Nuts
- **Seasoning:** Adobo, Black Pepper & Garlic Powder
- **Sauce:** Coconut & Liquid Aminos

## Chapter Conclusion

**The Buddha Bowl Blueprint can be used to create any vegan meal,** or any in general (although I recommend your meals be plant-based); whether that be a bowl, salad, or a plate of food.

**The ultimate goal with your nutrition is ensuring a proper balance of nutrients,** and this blueprint provides just that–complex carbs, lean protein, veggies, fruit, healthy fat, and all the micros in the world!

I love Buddha Bowls because there are endless combinations of what you can create and it's *never the same bite twice!* They're also quick and convenient, especially if you've already batch cooked a bunch of food. Simply go to your fridge, pick out a few (or all) of the foods you've prepared, portion them out, and then pop your dish in the microwave.

Once your food's heated (two to four minutes does the trick), add any fruit or raw veggies if you'd like, followed by some fats and seasoning, and then top it with a dressing or sauce and enjoy!

**Don't be afraid to try new things.** The worst that can happen is you end up not liking the combination of what you created, and that's okay! You know for next time. Have fun and keep experimenting! **You'll never know if you like something or not until you try it. ;)**

# Part 5

# Flexible Dieting

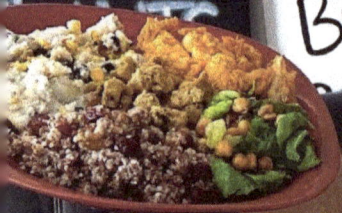

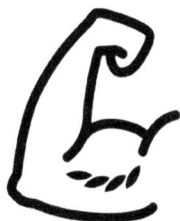

# Fad Diets

If I had a dollar for every fad diet, *"magic pill,"* or *"cleanse"* that I saw promising you to *"lose weight fast,"* I'd be a very rich man! Yeah, maybe you did have a great transformation after being on that protein-shake diet for a month, but what happened when you started eating real food again? My guess is you gained all of that weight back you just lost, if not more.

When it comes to losing weight, there are many ways to do so and do so rather fast. **But when it comes to building a healthy life with *results that last,* there is *no quick fix!***

**Dieting is about creating a *healthy* relationship with food;** and I use the terms *"diet"* and *"dieting"* very loosely because everyone has their own *"diet"* based on what they regularly eat. **A healthy relationship with food means:**
- Eliminating words such as *"cheats"* and *"treats"* when referring to food.
- Knowing the calories and macros of the food you regularly consume.
- Stressing less and understanding that **what matters most for the changes in your physique is *calories in versus calories burned* and *not* the exact food source.**

Doing so then allows you to consume *all* the foods you love, all the time, in healthy moderation. This is ***flexible dieting!***

Before we get into flexible dieting, I'm going to briefly overview a few of the most popular fad diets of today, some (or all) of which you may have tried at one point or another. The first is Atkins.

## Atkins

Popularized in 1972 with his book, *Dr. Atkins' Diet Revolution,* cardiologist Dr. Robert Atkins revolutionized the high-protein/low-carb weight-loss fad.

**The typical macros for the Atkins diet are:**
- **Carbs:** 10-20%
- **Protein:** 40-50%
- **Fat:** 40-50%

For these daily macro goals to be achieved, the Atkins diet promotes eating foods such as fatty meats, fish, butter, and cheese and says to avoid foods such as bananas, beans, grains, and potatoes. Nuts are allowed, and so are vegetables, but only if they're low in net carbs (the sum of total carbs minus fiber).

**When first adopting the Atkins diet, people will usually see rapid weight loss, but it's primarily due to three reasons–the first being the loss of water and glycogen.**

**Our body's primary source of fuel is glucose (carbs)**–the reason why we have such a large storage capacity for them.[7] **The average adult**

---

[7] See page 44.

**brain needs at least 130 grams of glucose per day alone to properly function.**

When your body stores carbs, it stores the glucose in your muscles and liver as glycogen. For every gram of glycogen stored, your body also stores three to four grams of water. Thus, **when you stop eating carbs, you deplete your glycogen stores, as well as your stored water. And so, not only do you lose the weight of the glycogen, but you also lose the water weight.**

**Second, when consuming a very low-carb diet, your body switches into a starvation mode known as ketosis and starts burning fat for fuel by producing chemicals called ketones.** Two of the main side effects of ketones are:

- **Nausea:** Nature's way of telling us we're eating poorly.
  - When you're nauseous, you tend to eat less and, thus, consume fewer calories, leading to more weight loss.
- **Diuresis:** More water (weight) loss.

Other common side effects include:

- Bad breath
- Constipation
- Fatigue
- Headache

**Third, because you're greatly restricted with what you can eat, often people following the Atkins diet will unconsciously eat less due to the severe lack of variety.** So, not only will your caloric intake be restricted from nausea, but boredom will also come into play. [20]

## Ketogenic

Low-carb on steroids, the ketogenic (keto) diet takes the low-carb diet to an even greater extreme.

**The typical macros for the Keto diet are:**
- **Carbs:** 5-10%
- **Protein:** 15-20%
- **Fat:** 75-80%

Just like those following Atkins, most people who try keto will lose significant weight initially for the same reasons, as well as fat for those who can stick it out long enough (so long as they're in a caloric deficit).

But when the sugar cravings start to hit (which they eventually do) and the willpower runs out (which it almost always does), these keto warriors go right back to stuffing their faces with whatever carbs they can find because they've been restricted from them for so long. This then leads to gaining all the weight back they just had lost–not because of the carbs, but because they're now consistently overeating.

## Paleo

The *"new-and-improved"* Atkins diet, the Paleo diet proclaims that the best way to eat is to eat only prehistoric foods; in other words, *"what the Neanderthal man would eat"*–even though his probable life expectancy was thirty years.

Foods to consume are the same as the Atkins diet, but the meat and fish should be *"pasture-raised,"* *"organic,"* or *"wild-caught"* (as if caveman hunted *"pasture-raised"* cattle). Bananas, dried fruit, and potatoes can also be eaten, as well (which is a big plus).

Nonetheless, beans, legumes, and wheat are strict forbidden–even though the healthiest and longest-lived cultures[8] in the world consume diets high in these foods. Other foods to avoid are those that are industrially processed, including cookies, dairy, donuts, white bread, etc.

What I like about the Paleo diet is its emphasis on the nutrient-density of what you're consuming, which makes you consider what your food actually is. Ironically, at the same time that the Paleo industry shuns processed food, it also produces its own processed forms of Paleo bread, cookies, and protein bars and claims them to be *"as functionally equivalent"* to what prehistoric man may have consumed– a little confusing and ridiculous if you ask me. [20]

**The typical macros for the Paleo diet are:**
- **Carbs:** 15-30%
- **Protein:** 20-30%
- **Fat:** 40-65%

## Weight Watchers

The most flexible of the four, Weight Watchers (WW) uses a point system called SmartPoints for tracking food. All food and beverages are assigned points based on their calories–the more calories the food or beverage contains, the more points it'll be. Depending on your weight and goals, WW provides you with daily and weekly SmartPoint targets that you must meet by tracking your food consumption.

There aren't any specific macro percentages to follow; and the best part about WW is that you're allowed to eat whatever you want, as long as you stay at or under your daily and weekly SmartPoint totals.

---

[8] See page 58.

The drawback to WW, however, is that there are over 200 *"zero-point"* foods that you don't need to track including beans, chicken breast, eggs, fish, and vegetables. Yet these foods all contain plenty of calories (aside from veggies); especially chicken breast, eggs, and fish.

Thus, if someone consumed all of their daily SmartPoints, in addition to unlimited untracked servings of chicken, eggs, and fish; undoubtedly, they wouldn't lose weight. It's also highly probable they'd gain weight instead, as they'll likely be in a caloric surplus. [40]

## Nutrient-Timing Myths

Lastly, we have the most common nutrient-timing myths. **Nutrient timing** is defined as *the time during the day for when it's best to eat certain nutrients.* Although none are named fad diets, they're all food myths that many people fall victim to daily. First up, we have breakfast.

### Breakfast

The long-standing belief about breakfast is that it's *"the most important meal of the day!"* But is it actually?

No, *actually it's not.* **No meal is *the most important;* instead, what's most important is *calories in versus calories burned* and the nutrient density of *all* of your meals.** So, whether you prefer to eat a large breakfast, a small one, or skip it altogether, what will ultimately determine your results is your caloric intake and the quality of your food.

There is some research that actually suggests that delaying your breakfast by intermittent fasting and eliminating simple carbs first thing in the morning will help stabilize your blood sugar levels, improve your body's ability to utilize sugar during the day, and allow your growth hormone (which is stimulated while you sleep) to reach its max peak after waking up. However, this research is still new and was done mostly on animal subjects with few conclusive human studies. [34]

## Dinner
With that being said, *it must be all about dinner then!*

Wrong again. No matter if you prefer to eat a small dinner or go to bed feeling full, caloric intake and food quality trump all.

## Carbs Before Bed
*What about carbs before bed? They make you fat, right?*

Nope. I eat carbs before bed all the time, and so can you! Plus, **carbs don't make you fat. *Overeating* makes you fat.**

## Meal Frequency
*Okay, okay, fine. But meal frequency definitely matters! I need to eat five to six small meals per day to speed up my metabolism because the Cosmopolitan told me to!*

Although this is something that I used to preach when I first started coaching (*face in palm*), this fallacy bears just as much relevancy as if I said that burning 100 calories while doing jumping jacks is better for you than burning 100 calories while riding a bike–*which it's not.*

***100 calories burned is 100 calories burned, it doesn't matter how you burned them!***

Your metabolism speeds up or down based on how high your activity level is, how much muscle mass you have, and how much you're eating. The higher your activity level, the more muscle mass you have, and the more calories you're taking in overall (especially in the form of carbs and protein); the faster your metabolism will be, and vice versa.

**Thus, if your daily fat-loss calorie goal is 2,000 calories, your body doesn't care if you eat five small meals of 400 calories each or only two big ones of 1,000 each. As long as you stay at or under your daily fat-loss goal, *you'll lose weight!***

**What will ultimately determine your physique goals is *calories in versus calories burned.***

- If you're consuming more than you're burning, then you'll gain weight.
- If you're consuming as much as you're burning, you'll stay the same.
- If you're consuming less than you're burning, then you'll lose weight.

**This is why *what* and *when* you're eating doesn't matter. As long as you're in a caloric deficit, *you'll lose weight,* if that's your goal.**

To prove this point, Mark Haub, a professor of nutrition at Kansas State, went on an extreme *"junk-food"* diet. For 10 weeks, two-thirds of his meals consisted of mainly Doritos, Little Debby Snack Cakes, Oreos, and Twinkies. He did eat some vegetables and took a daily multivitamin, as well, but ensured that he ate only a max of 1,800 calories per day.

The result? **After 10 weeks, he lost 27 pounds and reduced his body-fat percentage from 33% to 24%. Not only that, his bad cholesterol dropped by 20%, and his triglycerides dropped by 34%.**

I'm not saying, though, that you should start eating only chips and cookies to lose weight. If Professor Haub had continued with his junk-food diet long-term, there's no doubt he would have started to suffer from health issues due to a lack of nutrients and antioxidants. [20]

**Nonetheless, you can still eat chips, cookies, cake, ice cream, and whatever other junk food you please, regardless of your goals. But these foods should be consumed in *healthy moderation* where the majority of your diet is of nutrient-dense plant-based foods.**

This, my friends, is the **80|20 Rule.**

5.2

# 80|20 Rule

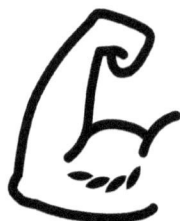

The first step to flexible dieting is subscribing to the **80|20 rule,** which says that **at least 80% of your diet should be filled with nutrient-dense foods and the other 20% can come from empty calories. Nutrient density** is defined as *a food's nutrient content, relative to its calories, based on the micronutrients (vitamins, minerals, and phytochemicals) that it provides to your body.*[9]

**The goal should be to meet your vitamin and mineral needs through your food consumption** that way you don't have to waste money on expensive vitamin and mineral supplements to make up for what your diet lacks.

Moreover, nutrient-dense foods (aka, *plants*) generally have far fewer calories per gram than their processed counterparts. Meaning, you can eat large portions without overeating in calories, resulting in you feeling full and satisfied for longer.

**The other 20% of your diet can then consist of foods that many would typically consider a** *"cheat"* **or** *"treat."* However, because we're eliminating these words from our food vocabulary, we'll instead refer to these foods as **empty calories:** *foods with low nutritional value that are*

---

[9] See the "Best Nutrient-Dense Foods" list, page 97.

*calorically dense; typically processed; and either very high in fat, preservatives, sodium, sugar, or all four.*[10]

Consuming empty calories (that are often viewed negatively when *"dieting"*) is perfectly okay because **your mental health is just as important as your physical health, and *even more important* than your outward appearance.**

If you're continually restricting yourself of the things you love, you won't be happy–*especially when it comes to food!* Instead of withholding entirely from the empty calories you enjoy eating, why not learn how to build them into your everyday diet in healthy moderation?

***What matters most is calories in versus calories burned.* So even if you were only to eat plain tofu and rice every day, you can still gain weight if you're overeating!**

This leads us to step two of flexible dieting: **calorie counting.**

---

[10] See the "Empty Calories" list, page 104.

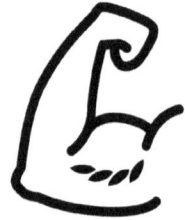

# Calorie Counting

*Calories in versus calories burned* **will ultimately determine the changes in your physique.** Therefore, to learn how to build a well-balanced sustainable diet without sacrificing your favorite foods, yet still reach your goals, calorie counting is the way to go.

## Calculating Your Calories

To determine your daily calories based on your goals, start by calculating your **Body-Weight Maintenance Calories (BWMC):** *the average daily number of calories required to maintain your current body weight,* by using your body weight (BW) and the chart below.

- **BWMC:** BW × Activity Multiplier

### BWMC Multipliers

| Lifestyle | Sedentary | Moderately Active | Active | Very Active |
|:---:|:---:|:---:|:---:|:---:|
| **Hours of Physical Activity\*/Week** | 0-1 | 2-4 | 5-7 | 8+ |
| **Multiplier** | 12-13 | 14-15 | 16-17 | 18-19 |

*\*Includes purposeful exercise and physically laborious jobs (construction, landscaping, nursing, serving, etc.). Does **not** include additional cardio (see page 249).*

Those who live more active lifestyles and have faster metabolisms will want to use a higher multiplier. Those who live more sedentary and have slower metabolisms will want to use a lower one. Please note, however, that these calculations are only rough estimates.

**To get a better idea of your Exact BWMC:**
- Calculate your calories using a multiplier that matches your activity level, and then accurately count your calories for two weeks consuming your **Calculated BWMC** on average every day.
- Weigh yourself at the beginning of the two weeks, each day during, and once more at the end. Ensure each weigh-in is at the same time every day (a total of 15 weigh-ins).
  - Ideally, you should weigh yourself while naked and in a fasted state, first thing in the morning after waking up and using the bathroom. Doing so will ensure the highest degree of accuracy and consistency.
- At the end of two weeks, compare your final weigh-in to your first.
  - If after two weeks your weight stayed the same, then your **Calculated BWMC** is accurate.
  - If your weight increased, then your **Exact BWMC** is less than what you initially calculated.
  - If your weight decreased, then it's higher.

**A pound equals 3,500 calories.**
- **If you gained weight,** subtract your *first weight* from your final weight, and then multiply that number by 3,500.
- **If you lost weight,** subtract your *final weight* from your first weight, and then multiply that number by 3,500.

This number represents your total caloric surplus or deficit over the two weeks. Therefore, if you gained one pound, then you ate an excess of

3,500 calories during those two weeks, and vice versa if you lost one pound.

**To determine your Exact BWMC,** divide your total two-week caloric surplus or deficit by 14. This will give you your average daily two-week surplus or deficit. You can then add or subtract this number, respectively, from your **Calculated BWMC** to get your **Exact BWMC.**

For example, Athlete #1 is trying to ensure the accuracy of his **Calculated BWMC.** At the beginning of the two weeks, he weighs himself first thing in the morning while naked and in a fasted state after using the bathroom. He weighs **175 pounds.** He lives an **active lifestyle** and, therefore, calculates his calories using **16 as his caloric multiplier,** making his **average daily caloric maintenance 2,800 calories.**

During the next two weeks, Athlete #1 eats an average of 2,800 calories each day and weighs himself every morning. After two weeks has passed, he records his **final weight check-in at 173 pounds.** He then reviews all of his weight check-ins over the last two weeks looking for large fluctuations, and there hasn't been any, as his weight consistently decreased. Meaning, his new weight of 173 is accurate, and he's actually **lost two pounds of fat.**

### Pro Tip
If there are large fluctuations in your daily weight check-ins when trying to determine your **Exact BWMC;** instead of solely comparing your final weight check-in to your first, use your two-week average weight instead.

**To calculate your two-week average weight**, add up all of your weigh-ins (not including your first, but including your last–14 total); and then divide that sum by 14 to get your average weight over the two weeks. Compare this average weight to your first weigh-in to see if you gained, maintained, or lost; and then use this number for the rest of your calculations.

Athlete #1 then multiplies two pounds by 3,500 calories to get 7,000, which tells him that he **ate at a deficit of 7,000 calories** over the last two weeks. **To determine his average daily two-week caloric deficit, he divides 7,000 by 14 to get 500.** He then adds 500 to his **Calculated BWMC** to make his **Exact BWMC 3,300 calories;** meaning his **actual maintenance caloric multiplier is closer to 19** and not 16. Refer to the calculations below.

**Exact BWMC Calculations for Athlete #1**
- **BW:** 175 lbs.
- **Lifestyle:** Active
- **Estimated Caloric Multiplier:** 16
- **Calculated BWMC:** 175 lbs. × 16 = 2,800 kcals
- **Final Weight After Two Weeks at BWMC:** 173 lbs.
- **Total Weight Lost:** 175 lbs. - 173 lbs. = 2 lbs.
- **Total Two-Week Caloric Deficit:** 2 lbs. × 3,500 kcals = 7,000 kcals
- **Average Daily Two-Week Caloric Deficit:** 7,000 kcals ÷ 14 days = 500 kcals
- **Exact BWMC:** 2,800 kcals + 500 kcals = 3,300 kcals
- **Actual Caloric Multiplier:** 3,300 kcals ÷ 175 lbs. = 18.86

Every person's body is unique, so trial and error will always come into play. **Once you know your Exact BWMC, add or subtract calories based on your goals.**
- **Muscle Gain:** Add
- **Fat Loss:** Subtract

Again, a pound equals 3,500 calories. Meaning, **to gain or lose a pound each week; you'd add or subtract, respectively, 500 calories from your BWMC.**

- 3,500 kcals ÷ 7 days/week = 500 kcals/day

**For muscle gain with minimal added fat, aim to gain 0.5-1 pounds per week (a 250-500 daily caloric surplus).** If gaining weight is all you care about and extra fat isn't a concern, consume as much as you'd like!

**For optimal fat burn with minimal muscle loss, aim to lose 0.5-2 pounds per week (a 250-1,000 daily caloric deficit), depending on your body-fat percentage (BFP).**

- The lower your BFP, the smaller your deficit should be.
- The higher your BFP, the greater your deficit can be.

### Ideal Daily Fat-Loss Deficit

| Male BFP* | Female BFP* | Daily Deficit (kcals) |
|:---:|:---:|:---:|
| > 40 | > 50 | 1,000+ |
| 25-40 | 35-50 | 750-1,000 |
| 10-25 | 20-35 | 500-750 |
| < 10 | < 20 | 250-500 |

*See the BFP Example Charts, page 165.*

However, just as eating less is necessary for burning fat, eating *enough* is equally important for proper bodily function, no matter your BFP. **Everyone** has a **Basal Metabolic Rate (BMR):** *the amount of energy required to maintain vital bodily functions (breathing, pulse, blood flow, etc.) while in a resting state (sleeping or lying still).*

- For American **men,** the average BMR is 1,800 kcals.
- For American **women,** it's 1,400 kcals. [7]

**To estimate your BMR, multiply your BW by 9 to 11.** The number you choose will be based on your current BFP.

### BMR Multipliers

| Male BFP* | Female BFP* | Multiplier |
|:---:|:---:|:---:|
| > 25 | > 30 | 9 |
| 15-25 | 20-30 | 10 |
| 10-15 | 15-20 | 10.5 |
| < 10 | < 15 | 11 |

*See the BFP Example Charts, page 165.*

To burn fat, you must eat less than you're burning. But if you consistently eat at too large of a deficit, three things will happen:

1. Your metabolism will slow because your body will go into starvation mode and try conserving whatever energy possible.
2. Your workout performance will decrease because you won't have enough energy to perform at your best resulting in fewer calories burned.
3. Your body will start burning its muscle mass, on top of its fat, because it needs the energy that you're restricting it from to function properly.

**When trying to lose weight, you don't want to feel like you're starving yourself. You want to have consumed enough food to be satiated, but not too much to ensure you're eating at a *controlled* caloric deficit.** This will ensure that you maintain your muscle mass, which will result in your body:

- Burning fat faster, as muscle requires more calories to sustain itself than fat does.
- Looking leaner at a higher BFP.

You also won't turn into a grumpy troll who's always in need of a Snicker's Bar... **Therefore, no matter how much fat you have to lose, *never eat less than your BMR!* It'll only hurt you in the long run.**

For example, let's say summer is right around the corner, and Athlete #1 wants to shed a few pounds of fat so that he looks his best while on the beach. Using his **Exact BWMC** of 3,300 calories that we calculated earlier; if Athlete #1 wants to lose a pound of fat per week, then he should consume an average of 2,800 calories per day. If he wants to lose two pounds of fat per week, then he should consume an average of 2,300 calories per day. Refer to the calculations below.

**Daily Fat-Loss Calories for Athlete #1**
- **Exact BWMC:** 3,300 kcals
- **Lose 1 lb./Week:** 3,300 kcals - 500 kcals = **2,800 kcals**
- **Lose 2 lbs./Week:** 3,300 kcals - 1,000 kcals = **2,300 kcals**

### Pro Tip

As your daily calorie goal is an *average* number that you should stick to each day, if on some days you want to eat more, then go ahead and do so. Just eat that much less the next day or few days.

For example, Athlete #1's average daily fat-loss calorie goal to lose one pound per week is 2,800 calories. If one day he's extra hungry and eats 3,400 calories (600 more than his average daily goal), then the next day he should eat only 2,200 (600 less than his average daily goal) to balance things out. Alternatively, he could eat only 2,500 calories for the next two (300 less than his average daily goal for two days–600 less in total); or even 2,600 for the next three (200 less than his average daily goal for three days).

To keep track of this while counting, rather than adding the surplus of 600 calories into the current day for when he ate the food, Athlete #1 would instead add the extra calories into his first meal of the following day. This way, when the next day comes, and he goes to log his food, he'll only have 2,200 calories left to use for that day out of his 2,800. Meaning, if he sticks to that 2,200 calories for the day, he'll be perfectly balanced out by day's end. He could also log 300 calories into his first meal for the next two days, which would leave him with 2,500 to eat each day.

Personally, I prefer the second and third options of eating only 300 calories less for two days or 200 less for three, rather than 600 less for one. Drastically going from very high calories one day to very little the next tends to backfire in the long run because it can easily lead to a cycle of yo-yo dieting and binging. As someone who's had much experience with periods of this personally, take it from me, *it's no fun!* But as always, to each his own. Choose whatever works best for *you.* **As long as you're eating at your calorie goal on an *average* daily basis, then you'll see the results you want!**

## Calculating Your Macros

To calculate your macros, you'll need three things:

1. Your **lean body weight (LBW):** *your body weight minus your body fat.*
2. Your average daily calorie goal.
3. The number of calories per gram for each macronutrient.

     o   **Protein:** 4 kcals/g
     o   **Carbs:** 4 kcals/g
     o   **Fat:** 9 kcals/g

## Protein Goal

The first macro to calculate is your protein, which will be determined by your **protein-goal range.**

### Protein-Goal Range

- 0.5-1.2 grams per pound of LBW

As you'll learn more about this in the "Macros, Micros, and More" section in *The Winner's Manual 2,* **the primary function of protein within the body is the maintenance and repair of muscle tissue. Therefore, to prevent muscle breakdown and ensure muscle protein synthesis** *(the growth of your muscles),* **you'll need to consume enough protein;** especially if you're consistently endurance and resistance training or dieting for fat loss.

**To calculate your LBW, you'll first need to determine your BFP.** If you've recently had this measured professionally through a Bod Pod, Dexa Scan, or Hydrostatic Weighing,[11] then use that measurement. If not, then use the respective male and female BFP example charts on the next page. Compare your current physique to the ones featured, then choose a percentage within the percentage range listed that corresponds to the physique you look closest to.

**Once you've determined your BFP, subtract it from 100% and then multiply that sum by your BW to calculate your LBW.** For example,

---

[11] See "Measuring Progress," page 266.

if Athlete #1 estimates that his current BFP is 10%, then his LBW would be 158 pounds.

**LBW Calculation for Athlete #1**
- **BFP:** 10%
- 100% - 10% = 90%
- 175 lbs. × 0.9 = 158 lbs.

| Male BFP Examples | Female BFP Examples |
|---|---|

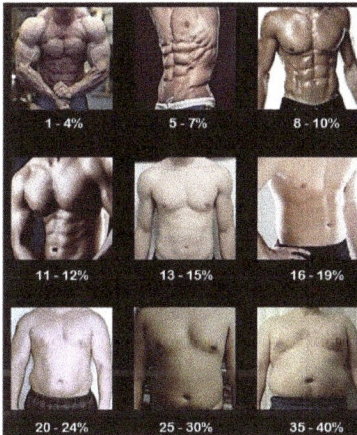

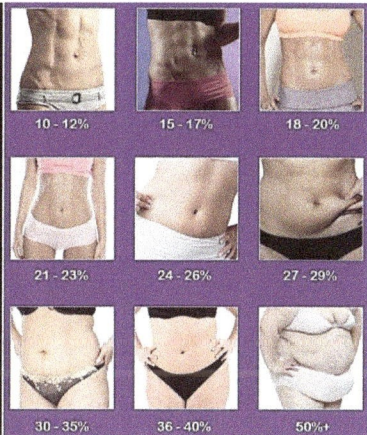

After calculating your LBW, **calculate the lower end of your protein-goal range by multiplying your LBW by 0.5 grams. Calculate the upper end by multiplying your LBW by 1.2 grams.**

For example, Athlete #1's LBW is 158 pounds. Therefore, his daily protein-goal range is 79-190 grams.

**Protein-Goal Range for Athlete #1**
- 158 lbs. × 0.5 g = 79 g

- 158 lbs. × 1.2 g = 190 g

Select a number within that range based on your activity level, goals, and personal preference.

### Ideal Protein-Goal Range

| Lifestyle | Sedentary | Moderately Active | Active | Very Active |
|---|---|---|---|---|
| **Hours of Physical Activity\*/Week** | 0-1 | 2-4 | 5-7 | 8+ |
| **Protein Goal\*\* (Gain/Maintain)** | 0.5-0.8 | 0.5-0.8 | 0.8-1 | 0.8-1 |
| **Protein Goal\*\* (Fat Loss)** | 0.8-1 | 0.8-1 | 1-1.2 | 1-1.2 |

*\*Includes purposeful exercise and physically laborious jobs (construction, landscaping, nursing, serving, etc.). \*\*Protein goals listed in g/lb. of LBW.*

**You'll want to choose a higher number if you:**
- Are a strength or endurance athlete (football player, marathoner, etc.).
- Live an active lifestyle (regular hiking, biking, skiing, swimming, etc.).
- Have an active job (construction, landscaping, nursing, serving, etc.).
- Have a goal of fat loss or muscle gain.
- Tend to eat more protein.

**You'll want to choose a lower one if you:**
- Live more sedentary.
- Have a goal of general health and maintenance.
- Tend to eat less protein.

## Fat Goal

The next macro to calculate is your fat. **For proper hormone regulation, it's best to consume no less than 0.3 grams of fat per pound of LBW.** Therefore, to calculate your daily fat requirement, multiply your LBW by 0.3 and 0.7. This will give you your **fat-goal range.**

**Fat-Goal Range**

- LBW × 0.30-0.70 g

Again, select a number within that range based on your personal preference. **If you tend to prefer less fat and more carbs, then you'll want to choose a lower number within that range. If you tend to eat less carbs and more fat, then you'll want to choose a higher one.** For example, Athlete #1's LBW is 158 pounds. Therefore, his daily fat-goal range is 47-111 grams.

**Fat-Goal Range Calculations for Athlete #1**

- 158 lbs. × 0.3 = 47 g
- 158 lbs. × 0.7 = 111 g

## Carbohydrate Goal

Once you know your protein and fat goals, your carbs will fill in the rest. To calculate your carb goal, take your daily caloric requirement and subtract both the number of calories you're consuming in protein and fat; then divide that number by four. This will give you your daily **carb goal** in grams.

**Daily Carb-Goal Calculation**

- **Protein Calories**: Protein Goal (g) × 4 kcals/g
- **Fat Calories:** Fat Goal (g) × 9 kcals/g
- **Carb Goal (g):** (Daily Calories - Protein Calories - Fat Calories) ÷ 4 kcals/g

**Fiber Goal**

To aid with proper digestion, waste removal, and natural body detoxification, consume at least 30-40 grams of fiber per day. **If your goal is fat loss, then the more fiber the better because it'll keep you fuller for longer without adding calories, as most fiber calories aren't absorbed by the body.** Personally, I eat upwards of 50-70 grams of fiber per day.

For example, Athlete #1 is a strength athlete who lives a very active lifestyle and tends to eat more carbs and less fat. His current goal is fat loss. Therefore, he chooses to consume 1.2 grams of protein per pound of LBW and 0.3 grams of fat. Thus, his macro goals are 190 grams of protein, 47 grams of fat, and 404 grams of carbs (at least 30-40 of which is fiber).

**Macro-Goal Calculations for Athlete #1**
- **Fat-Loss Calorie Goal:** 2,800 kcals
- **Protein:** 158 lbs. × 1.2 g = **190 g** × 4 kcals/g = 760 kcals
- **Fat:** 158 lbs. × 0.3 g = **47 g** × 9 kcals/g = 423 kcals
- **Carbs:** (2,800 kcals - 760 kcals protein - 423 kcals fat) = 1,617 kcals ÷ 4 kcals/g = **404 g**
  - **Fiber ≥ 30-40 g**

These are the macros that Athlete #1 should consume on an average daily basis to burn one pound of fat per week.

## Macro Percentages Alternative

If you'd prefer an easier alternative for determining your macros; then select them from the percentage ranges below, multiply each by your daily calorie goal, and divide the sums by their respective number of calories per gram. Again, your choices will be made based on your goals and personal preference.

**Macro-Percentage Ranges for a Well-Balanced Diet**
- **Carbs:** 30-70%
- **Protein:** 15-35%
- **Fat:** 15-35%

For example, Athlete #1 decides to determine his macros using the percentage ranges, instead, and chooses them to be 60% carbs, 25% protein, and 15% fat. Therefore, his macros in grams are 420 grams of carbs, 175 grams of protein, and 47 grams of fat.

**Macro-Percentage Goal Calculations for Athlete #1**
- **Fat-Loss Calorie Goal:** 2,800 kcals
- **Carbs:** 2,800 kcals × 0.6 = 1,680 kcals ÷ 4 kcals/g = **420 g**
- **Protein:** 2,800 kcals × 0.25 = 700 kcals ÷ 4 kcals/g = **175 g**
- **Fat:** 2,800 kcals × 0.15 = 420 kcals ÷ 9 kcals/g = **47 g**

**No matter what macros you choose, at the end of the day,** *what's most important is your caloric and protein intake.*

If you're dieting for a fitness competition, then I'd recommend staying as close to your macro goals as possible, especially if you're working with a coach. **But if you don't have a specific event that you're preparing for, and you'd rather not be super strict on macros, focus instead on:**
- Consuming plenty of nutrient-dense foods.[12]
- Staying at or under your daily calorie goal and within your protein-goal range.
- Letting your carbs and fats fill in themselves based on whatever you're eating for that day.

---

[12] See the "Best Nutrient-Dense Foods" list, page 97.

Some days you'll crave more carbs, so go ahead and eat more; just counter by eating less fat. Other days you might want more fat, so eat fewer carbs. Remember, this is *flexible dieting.* No two days will be the same–unless, of course, you choose to eat the same thing every day… **Eat plenty of delicious and nutritious food, stick to your calorie and protein goals, and you'll be golden!**

## Counting Your Calories *(Accurately)*

Now that you know how to calculate your own calories and macros, the next step is tracking your food intake–*accurately.* How do you do this?

- First, **download MyFitnessPal** on your phone or tablet.
- Second, **buy a digital food scale and measuring cups** *(if you don't already own them).*
- Third, **measure or weigh all of the food you eat** *before* you **eat it.**

If you've never counted calories before, chances are you won't be the best at eyeballing and estimating serving sizes; meaning, the serving sizes you'll likely be logging won't be accurate. **Inaccurate serving sizes mean either too many or too little calories accounted for.** Multiply these inaccuracies times all of your meals for the day, and you could be either way under or way over your daily caloric total. **Always being too far under or too far over your daily calories will negatively affect you reaching your goals.**

Now, I know having to measure or weigh all of your food may seem like a pain at first because it adds extra time to your food preparation; but I guarantee *it's 100% worth it!*

## Using MyFitnessPal

Once you've downloaded MyFitnessPal (MFP), it'll give you calorie and macro goals based your information provided during the set-up process. You may use these if you wish, but I recommend using the numbers you calculated yourself (or were given by your coach).

**To manually enter your custom nutrition goals from the app dashboard:**

- Click *"More"* > *"Goals"* > *"Calorie & Macronutrient Goals"*

Once the **Calories & Macros** page opens, click *"Calories,"* input your calorie goal, and then click the checkmark in the top right-hand corner of the number pad.

For your macros, use the macro-percentage spin wheels to adjust the macros shown until they match your goals, or come as close as possible to them. If you're using the Premium version of MFP, then you can instead enter your exact macro goals in grams. Click the checkmark in the right-hand corner when finished.

## Adding Food to Your Diary

The first way to add food to your diary is by using the **barcode scanner.** This allows you to take a food package and scan the barcode to pull up the nutritional info right in the app. **To find the scanner, go to your Diary, select *"+ Add Food,"* and then click the barcode button in the top right corner.** Allow the app access to your camera.

The second way is to use the *"Search for a food"* option to search the app's database. **Simply type in the name and brand name of the food you'd like to add and hit *"Search."*** Usually, several options will appear, so you'll have to scroll through until you find the correct one.

How do you know when you've found the correct option? **Compare the nutrition facts in the app to those from the nutrition fact label on the food's packaging.**[13] If you're unable to find a matching option, then you can manually enter in the nutritional info yourself by creating a food.

# Nutrition Facts

Serving Size 2 tbsp. (33 g)
Servings Per Container 7

Amount Per Serving

**Calories** 20      Calories from Fat 10

% Daily Value*

## Creating a Food

**To manually enter nutritional info, click** *"+ Add Food,"* **scroll to the very bottom, and then select** *"Create a Food."* Type in the **Brand Name,** the **Description of the food,** the **Serving Size,** and enter in the **Servings per container** as *"1."*

**For the Serving Size, use ounces (oz.), grams (g), or milliliters (mL), as these will ensure the highest accuracy.** No matter if the serving size of the food is given in ounces or not, there's usually always a gram (or milliliter if a liquid) equivalent listed, as well. Use that.

### Pro Tip

If you're measuring a liquid, but your food scale doesn't have a milliliter option, one milliliter of liquid equates to one gram in

---

[13] Be aware of the food's state for which you're consuming it in. The same food raw (uncooked) will usually yield different calorie and macro totals than when cooked, and vice versa. See "Cooked vs. Uncooked Calories," page 195.

weight (1 mL = 1 g), so you may use the gram option instead. For example, one cup of liquid (240 milliliters) equals 240 grams when weighed.

If your food doesn't have a nutritional label (like raw fruit and veggies), then search the app using the name of the item with *"USDA"* at the end and look for the USDA options listed. Alternatively, you can use **acaloriecounter.com** to search the USDA database and then manually enter the information into MFP by creating a food. Typically, both *"raw"* and *"cooked"* options will be listed. Choose the one that corresponds to the state for which you'll be eating that food.

## How to Weigh Your Food

1. Turn on your food scale.
2. Place your empty bowl, cup, or plate on top.
3. **Tare**[14] the scale to bring it to zero.

---

[14] Tare weight represents the empty weight of an object. By hitting tare on your food scale after you've placed your plate or bowl on top, it'll zero out its weight so that only the weight of what you put on or inside it will appear.

4. Set the **serving size** of the food to be recorded in **MFP** to either **ounces (oz.), grams (g), or milliliters (mL).**
   o Ensure that this setting is either *"1 oz.," "1 g," or "1 mL."*
5. Set the scale's **units** to either **ounces (oz.), grams (g), or milliliters (mL)** to match the serving size in MFP.
6. Add the first ingredient of your meal to your dish.
7. Adjust the number of servings in MFP to match the weight on the scale.
8. Click the ✓ button in the top right corner of the app and then search for your next food.
9. Leave your first ingredient in or on your dish, and then **repeat** steps three through nine until you're finished logging all of your food for that meal.

For example, tonight you're making tofu for dinner with red potatoes, asparagus, and avocado. Once you've cooked your food and it comes time to weigh portions, turn on your food scale, and place your plate on top. Hit tare to zero out the scale and then add the tofu to your plate. Use your *"cooked"* tofu option and accurately log the tofu into MFP. Leave the tofu on the plate and then hit tare again to re-zero the weight. Add your potatoes and accurately record your *"cooked"* red potato serving. Tare the scale once more, then do the same for your asparagus and avocado.

### My Suggestion
Store your food scale on the counter so that it's always readily available to use. After some time, weighing your food and counting your calories will become routine. **Stick with it, and I guarantee you'll slowly start to see the results you've always wanted!**

## Tracking Homemade Dishes

When preparing meals at home using multiple ingredients, this is where it gets trickier to track, especially when the dish is divided among many people. *But have no fear!* Where there's a will, there's a way; and there most certainly is a way to track your homemade delights!

First, create a meal consisting of the raw ingredients for the dish. To do this, starting from the app dashboard:

- Click *"More"* > *"Meals, Recipes & Foods"* > *"Meals"* > *"Create a Meal"*

Name your meal whatever you'd like, click *"Add Food";* and then add all the raw ingredients for your dish, ensuring that you accurately enter the serving size for the amount of each used. Once you've added everything, click *"Save"* in the top right-hand corner to save your meal.

Notice that, as you add ingredients to your meal, the app provides you with the nutrition facts for everything combined. *This is key.* In your phone Notes or on a piece of paper, jot down the total calories and macros given for your meal with all of its ingredients, as you'll be referring back to them in a minute.

Once you've saved your meal and have recorded its calories and macros, go ahead and cook your dish. After your dish is finished cooking, place an empty bowl or plate on top of your food scale; set it to grams (g), zero it out, and transfer your food to that bowl or plate. The number that appears on the scale in grams will represent the total *"cooked"* serving size for your homemade dish. Jot this number down, as well.

Next, go back to the *"Meals, Recipes & Foods"* tab:

- Click *"Foods"* > *"Create a Food."*
- Enter in the **Brand Name** as *"Homemade."*

- Enter the **Description** as the same name for which you called your dish when creating a meal.
- Enter the **Serving Size** as its total *"cooked"* weight in grams.
- Enter the **Servings per container** as *"1."*
- Enter the **Nutrition Facts** using the calories and macros that you jotted down earlier after creating a meal with the dishes' raw ingredients.
- Click the ✓ button in the top right-hand corner to save your food.

Now, you have both an accurate serving size for your cooked homemade dish in grams per its total weight, along with precise calorie and macro totals. To add your portion in, simply add it as you would any other food.

- Go to the meal in your diary for which you would like to add your food to.
- Click *"+Add Food"* > *"My Foods."*
- Select your homemade dish.
- Set the **Serving Size** to *"1 gram."*
- Weigh your portion in grams.
- Adjust the number of **Servings** to match your portion.

*And bam! You just accurately tracked your homemade dish!*

## Caloric Accuracy Check

Often, food producers will round the number of calories listed on their nutritional labels to the nearest interval of five or ten for ease of reading. Because of this, the number of calories you've consumed according to MFP will usually be slightly off. To check if the calories you've consumed are actually what the app says, crosscheck them by multiplying your macronutrients.

For example, in my diary below, it says that I've consumed 2,011 calories (*"Food"*) and that I have 389 calories *"Remaining"* to meet my daily goal. To check if this is accurate or not, I'll scroll to the very bottom of my dairy, click *"Nutrition,"* and then *"Nutrients."* This will pull up an overview of the nutrients I've consumed for that day.

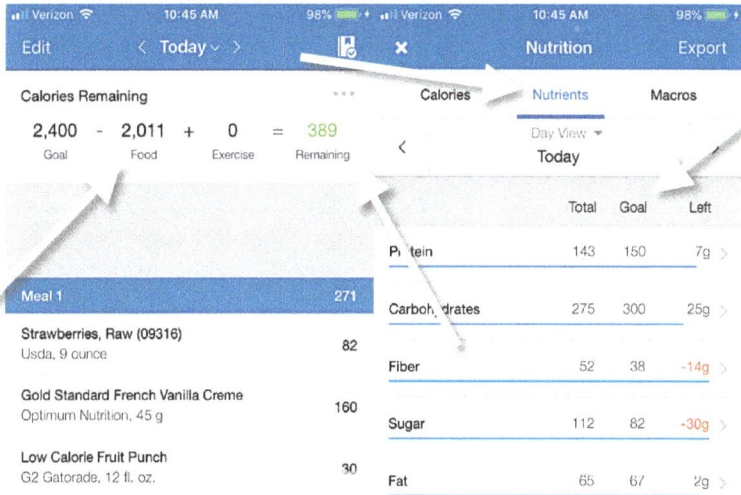

| | Total | Goal | Left |
|---|---|---|---|
| Protein | 143 | 150 | 7g > |
| Carbohydrates | 275 | 300 | 25g > |
| Fiber | 52 | 38 | -14g > |
| Sugar | 112 | 82 | -30g > |
| Fat | 65 | 67 | 2g > |

Calories Remaining

2,400 − 2,011 + 0 = 389
Goal    Food    Exercise   Remaining

Meal 1                                        271

Strawberries, Raw (09316)                      82
Usda, 9 ounce

Gold Standard French Vanilla Creme            160
Optimum Nutrition, 45 g

Low Calorie Fruit Punch                        30
G2 Gatorade, 12 fl. oz.

I'll then multiply each of the macros listed in the *"Total"* column by their respective number of calories per gram and add their sums together. This will give me the actual number of calories I've consumed for that day. I can then subtract this number from my daily goal to determine how many calories I still have left.

## Actual Calories Consumed Based on Macros
- **Protein:** 143 g × 4 kcals/g = 572 kcals
- **Carbs:** 275 g × 4 kcals/g = 1,100 kcals
- **Fat:** 65 g × 9 kcals/g = 585 kcals
- **Total Calories Consumed (kcals):** 572 + 1,100 + 585 = **2,257**

- **Total Calories Remaining (kcals):** 2,400 - 2,257 = **143**
- **Caloric Inaccuracy (kcals):** 389 - 143 = **246**

Now I know a difference of 246 calories may not seem like a whole lot, but over time those calories add up. **If you're consuming an additional 250 calories more than what you thought you were every day,** *that's an additional 1,750 extra calories per week!* If your goal is fat loss, but your results are slower than what you expected, this could be why. To avoid this, simply crosscheck your macros and you'll be good.

## Chapter Conclusion

Calorie counting is the *best* tool for flexible dieting because it's a free education on food. By tracking your food intake regularly:

1. You learn the calorie and macro profiles of everything you eat.
2. You see what, and precisely *how much,* you're consuming.

Knowing this information is important because **what matters most for the changes in your physique is** *calories in versus calories burned.* Counting gives you peace of mind that you're consuming the right number of calories to reach your goals while still enjoying all the foods you love in healthy moderation.

**5.4**

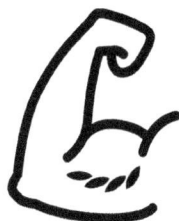

# Meal Prepping

The beauty of batch cooking and calorie counting is flexibility. However, if you prefer more structure to your diet, then I highly recommend meal prepping, especially if you're busy and always on-the-go.

**Having all of your meals planned and prepared ahead of time takes away the worry of what your next meal's going to be and allows you to focus fully on your work/life tasks at hand.**

**Meal prepping is also very helpful if you're preparing for a fitness competition or even personal events like a pool party or wedding.** During the final weeks of prep, your BFP will be very low, and the slightest fluctuations in what you're eating can significantly alter the appearance of your physique. Not only does meal prepping protect against this, but it ensures that you stay on track and *crush your goals!*

## Steps to Meal Prepping

### 1.  Determine Your Number of Meals per Day

Many people prefer to eat the standard three meals per day. Others prefer to eat breakfast, lunch, and dinner; but also like to have a snack between each meal. Some even prefer to eat only one to two large meals, and that's it. Choose whatever works best for *you.*

## 2.  Determine the Number of Days for Your Plan

Some people like to plan for the whole week; some for three days at a time. Others prefer prepping for the weekdays (Monday through Friday) when they're busiest and need the most structure; then leave the weekends open for when they have more time to eat freely. As always, do whatever works best for *you*.

## 3.  Calculate Your Calories

For simplicity, evenly distribute your calories among your desired number of meals. Thus, if your daily fat-loss calorie goal is 2,100, and you prefer eating three meals per day, then each meal should contain 700 calories.

### Pro Tip

If you like having your three main meals each day, but also like to have dessert at night after dinner, then I recommend dividing your calories into four meals and making the fourth meal (your dessert) be half the size of your three main ones. For example, if sticking to 2,100 calories: instead of having three 700-calorie meals, have three 600-calorie main ones (1,800 total); which leaves you with 300 calories leftover for dessert.

## 4.  Set Your Macros

If you calculated your macros based on personal preference and you know their values in grams, then divide each of your daily macro goals by your desired number of meals. For example, if your daily macros in grams are 270 carbs, 150 protein, and 45 fat, then your macros per meal should be 90 carbs, 50 protein, and 15 fat.

- **Carbs:** 270 g ÷ 3 meals = **90 g**
- **Protein:** 150 g ÷ 3 meals = **50 g**
- **Fat:** 47 g ÷ 3 meals = **15 g**

If you determined your daily macros based on percentages, then multiply each macro goal by your allotted number of calories per meal; then divide the sums by their respective number of calories per gram, to determine your macros per meal. For example, if your macro-percentage goal is 50% carbs, 25% protein, and 25% fat, and your calories-per-meal goal is 700, then your macros per meal in grams should be 88 carbs, 44 protein, and 19 fat.

- **Carbs:** 700 kcals × 0.5 = 350 kcals ÷ 4 kcals/g = **88 g**
- **Protein:** 700 kcals × 0.25 = 175 kcals ÷ 4 kcals/g = **44 g**
- **Fat:** 700 kcals × 0.25 = 175 kcals ÷ 9 kcals/g = **19 g**

## 5.  Choose Your Food

Once you've determined your calories and macros per meal, you'll next want to decide what to eat. Choose a few of your favorite nutrient-dense foods[15] per each macro and mix and match them to create your meals.

For example, your food choices could be:

- **Carbs, Fruit & Veggies:** Sweet potato, quinoa, broccoli, Brussels sprouts, oatmeal, and banana.
- **Protein:** Seitan, mock meat, and protein powder.
- **Fat:** Avocado, dressing, and peanut butter.

## 6.  Calculate Your Meal Portions

To calculate your portions per meal, use MFP to adjust the serving size of each food until, together, they total your desired macro goals for the meal you'll be consuming them. Don't worry about being super precise with each macro, just stay as close to your goals as possible.

---

[15] See the "Best Nutrient-Dense Foods" list, page 97.

### 7.  Buy Your Food

After your meal plan is set, multiply each serving of food by the number of days you'll be following it, then buy that amount of each food when you go shopping. For example, if you were planning on following the sample lunch plan on the next page for three days, then you'd buy:

- **Sweet Potato:** 24 oz. (8 oz. × 3)
- **Seitan:** 390 g (130 g × 3) (This is how much you'd make if it's homemade)
- **Broccoli:** 24 oz. (8 oz. × 3)
- **Avocado:** 9 oz. (3 oz. × 3)
- **Tomato Basil Dressing:** 3 oz. (1 oz. × 3) (Obviously you wouldn't buy just three ounces of dressing, you'd buy the whole bottle. But for the purpose of the example, three ounces is what you'd use in total.)

### 8.  Cook

Lastly, once you've completed every step above, it's time to start cooking! Follow the **Steps to Batch Cooking** (page 126) and cook everything in your plan or seek out a meal prep company to have your meals made for you. If you don't want to prepare all of your meals ahead of time, that's okay. At least you've already planned them out. That way, when your next meal comes, there's no thinking necessary–*you already know what you're having!*

## Sample Meal Prep

Daily Calories & Macros

- **Calories:** 2,100
- **Carbs:** 270 g
- **Protein:** 150 g
- **Fat:** 45 g

Calories & Macros Per Meal
- **Calories:** 700
- **Carbs:** 90 g
- **Protein:** 50 g
- **Fat:** 15 g

Food Choices
- **Carbs, Fruit & Veggies:** Sweet potato, quinoa, broccoli, Brussels sprouts, oatmeal, banana
- **Protein:** Seitan, beefless crumbles, protein powder
- **Fat:** Avocado, dressing, peanut butter

Meal Plan

### Breakfast

| Serving | Food | Calories | Carbs | Protein | Fat |
|---------|------|----------|-------|---------|-----|
| 80 g | Quaker Quick Oats | 310 | 54 | 10 | 6 |
| 4 oz. | Banana | 115 | 26 | 1 | 0.5 |
| 56 g | PEScience Vegan Protein Powder | 175 | 4 | 40 | 0 |
| 16 g | Peanut Butter | 95 | 5.5 | 3 | 7 |
| | Total | 695 | 89.5 | 54 | 13.5 |

### Lunch

| Serving | Food | Calories | Carbs | Protein | Fat |
|---------|------|----------|-------|---------|-----|
| 8 oz. | Sweet Potato | 225 | 48 | 8 | 0 |
| 130 g | Seitan | 180 | 10 | 35 | 0 |
| 8 oz. | Broccoli | 90 | 16 | 6.5 | 0 |
| 3 oz. | Avocado | 155 | 7 | 2 | 13 |
| 1 oz. | Tomato Basil Dressing | 55 | 2 | 0 | 5 |
| | Total | 705 | 83 | 51.5 | 18 |

## Dinner

| Serving | Food | Calories | Carbs | Protein | Fat |
|---------|------|----------|-------|---------|-----|
| 200 g | Quinoa | 345 | 56.5 | 16.5 | 6 |
| 150 g | Gardein Beefless Crumbles | 220 | 15.5 | 31 | 3.5 |
| 8 oz. | Brussels Sprouts | 85 | 12 | 9 | 0 |
| 1 oz. | Sesame Ginger Dressing | 55 | 7 | 1 | 2.5 |
| | Total | 705 | 91 | 57.5 | 12 |

## Calorie & Macro Totals

| Calories | Carbs (g) | Protein (g) | Fat (g) |
|----------|-----------|-------------|---------|
| 2,105 | 263.5 | 163 | 43.5 |

*Macros are listed in grams (g) and are rounded to the nearest ½ gram. Calories are rounded to the nearest interval of five.*

**If you'd prefer not to eat the exact same meals every day, try creating two or three plans to rotate through with different food choices.** This will make the meal prepping process longer and more tedious, however, as you'll have more food to cook. In this case, seeking out a local meal prep company might be best if you'd like a rotating plan but don't want to spend the extra time cooking.

**Another great option for variety is to keep the same food choices but vary how you mix them per meal. You can also use a different dressing or topping, as well, to change each meal's overall flavor.**

For example, instead of eating quinoa, beefless crumbles, and Brussels sprouts with sesame ginger dressing every night for dinner; use a Thai peanut dressing every other night, instead. You can also mix your food choices and create new combinations, like quinoa with sweet potatoes, broccoli, beefless crumbles, and avocado, all topped with a low-calorie BBQ sauce–my favorite is **Stubb's Sticky Sweet.**

## Chapter Conclusion

**If you're really serious about reaching your goals and maintaining your results, then meal prepping can be a *huge* help.** Use it when you need to, and don't be afraid to have fun experimenting when creating your meals. Again, *you'll never know if you like something or not until you try it.* ;)

# Common Food Mistakes

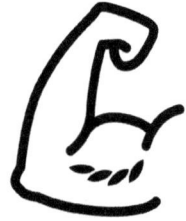

Was there ever a time where you thought you were eating really *"clean"* and yet you still didn't see the results in your physique that you wanted?

Trust me, I've been there, too.

In this chapter, I'm going to cover the most common food mistakes that I see many people make. These mistakes are ones that I'd regularly make myself and are typically the culprit of stagnant results–all of which can be revealed through accurately counting. The first is caloric drinks.

## Caloric Drinks

Liquid calories are easily one of the main reasons why so many people struggle to lose weight. Why?

Because **when you drink caloric drinks, your body doesn't register those calories.** What I mean by that is, **when you drink any liquid that has calories, your body will still require solid food to keep it satiated.** So, even though you may have just consumed 200 calories worth of orange juice, it was only 200 calories worth of a liquid. You'll have to consume more solid calories to feel full, only increasing your caloric intake for that day.

For example, in 12 ounces of Pepsi, there are 150 calories and 41 grams of sugar. **If your daily caloric maintenance requirement is 2,000** calories and you drink three 12-ounce cans, *that's 420 calories and 120 grams of sugar!* This means you're already almost a fourth of the way to your calorie goal from just liquids, which do nothing for satiation. **Now tack on the calories from the meal you likely ate with those cans of soda, and you could have easily reached your daily goal in only one sitting!**

*"Well Bobby, I don't drink soda, I only drink juice, and that's so much better for you. Right?"*

***Wrong!***

In 8 ounces of Welch's 100% Grape Juice (yes, 8 ounces and not 12), there are 140 calories and 36 grams of sugar. This means that in 12 ounces, there are *210 calories and 54 grams of sugar!* **That's 60 more calories and 13 more grams of sugar in the 12-ounce grape juice equivalent of Pepsi, even though most people would consider grape juice to be** *"better"* **for you.**

If you're one of those people, don't feel bad because I used to be of that mindset too. Instead of getting a soda, I'd get juice thinking I was making a *"healthier"* decision when in reality my *"healthier"* choice was actually worse. To help illustrate this point, the table on the next page compares seven caloric drinks standard in the American diet.

As you can see, the *"healthiest"* of these drinks, in terms of the least amount of sugar, is milk. This (combined with its protein and calcium benefits) along with the dairy industry's drive to make money, is the reason why it's continuously pushed on us as a *"necessary"* part of our daily diet.

### Caloric Drinks Standard in the American Diet

|  | Brand | Calories | Fat | Carbs | Sugar | Protein |
|---|---|---|---|---|---|---|
| Soda | Pepsi | 100 | 0 | 28 | **28** | 0 |
| Grape Juice | Welch's | 140 | 0 | 36 | **36** | 0 |
| Lemonade | Brisk | 100 | 0 | 27 | **27** | 0 |
| Orange Juice | Tropicana | 110 | 0 | 26 | **22** | 2 |
| Iced Tea | Brisk | 50 | 0 | 15 | **15** | 0 |
| Sports Drink | Gatorade | 55 | 0 | 15 | **15** | 0 |
| 1% Milk | Hood | 110 | 2.5 | 13 | **12** | 8 |

*Serving size = 8 oz. Macronutrients listed in grams (g).*

**The reality is, though, humans don't need milk past infancy, much less that of another species.** Not only are humans the only species that drinks milk into adulthood, but we're also the only species to drink another species' milk.

**Cow's milk was designed for calves, and once those calves are weaned, they never drink milk again.** Could you imagine sitting down for dinner and pouring yourself a glass of your mother's breast milk? *I didn't think so.*

**If you're looking for an excellent source of calcium without the extra calories, sugar, and cow hormones, then give a plant or nut milk a try like almond milk.**[16] **In an eight-ounce serving of Silk's Unsweetened Almond Milk, there's *50% more calcium* than in the dairy-milk equivalent.** Plus, there are only 30 calories per serving, as opposed to 110. *You can't beat that!*

---

[16] See the "Best Nutrient-Dense Liquids" list, page 102.

## Oil & Butter

How often do you use oil when you cook? Whether it's canola, vegetable, olive, or coconut oil. Once a day?

My guess, if I were on stage speaking to an audience right now, at least 50% or more would have a hand raised. But why is cooking with oil considered a mistake you might ask, especially if it's with one of the healthy staples like olive or coconut oil? That, my friends, is revealed in the macros.

The macro profile of all four of these oils, including the *"healthy"* ones, is 120 calories, 14 grams of fat, zero grams of carbs, and zero grams of protein per tablespoon. **One tablespoon equals half an ounce, meaning that in one ounce of oil, there are 28 grams of fat and 240 calories–*in only one ounce!*** [1] So many calories in such a small amount of oil.

Let's say you just cooked yourself a nice healthy dinner, which consisted of six ounces each of broccoli, Seitan, and sweet potato, plus three ounces of avocado. Assuming no additional sauces or dressings, your calorie and macro totals for this meal would come to 620 calories, 58 grams of protein, 68 grams of carbs, and 13 grams of fat.

Now, pretend you sautéed your broccoli using one tablespoon of olive oil, and roasted your sweet potatoes using another. **Your total calories for this meal just went from 620 to *860,* and your total grams of fat just went from 13 to *41! Talk about hidden calories!***

**The other problem with cooking with oil is that when it's heated, it oxidizes, meaning, it digests for you. And so, if you consume this**

oil with other food, your body will burn the other food, first, and the oil will go straight to your fat cells, instead.

Yes, olive oil does indeed have a few positive health benefits–antioxidants and monounsaturated fats. But there are many other foods to choose from[17] that provide those same antioxidants and unsaturated fats. Ones that are much more voluminous and will actually keep you full–**avocado and nuts of all sorts to name a few.**

This goes for butter, too. The macro profile for one ounce of butter is 210 calories, 23 grams of fat, zero carbs, and zero protein. [1] Plus, butter isn't vegan and so if you're vegan, then it's something you definitely shouldn't consume.

### Oil & Butter Substitutes

Instead of using oil or butter when if you're baking, use a non-stick sheet liner, such as **Reynolds' Non-Stick Aluminum Foil,** and add water (if needed) to keep your food moist. **If you're sautéing or cooking on the stove, use only water, soy sauce, liquid aminos, or vinegar or lightly coat the pan with a non-stick spray.** There are also many non-stick baking sheets and pans on the market to purchase for use, as well.

If you'd still prefer to use oil, that's okay. **Be mindful of how much you're using and just like drinking caloric drinks, *cooking with oil is only a mistake if you're not adding the oil into your daily calories.***

## Dressings & Marinades

The mistake with dressings and marinades is the same as cooking with oil. Most are very high in fat because of their oil content, and they usually

---

[17] See the "Best Nutrient-Dense Fats" list, page 101.

have **10-14 grams of fat per two-tablespoon serving.**

**The typical serving size for dressings at restaurants is two to three ounces, which is four to six tablespoons in total.** Let's say you were at the 99 Restaurant and, for an appetizer, you ordered a garden salad with honey mustard dressing. The 99's Garden Salad consists of lettuce, tomatoes, cucumbers, roasted red peppers, Parmesan cheese, and croutons. Without dressing, it's only 120 calories.[18]

**In a two-ounce side of 99's Honey Mustard Dressing, there are 340 calories, 0 grams of protein, 10 grams of carbs, and *34 grams of fat!*** That means if you add just two ounces of honey mustard to your salad, then 75% of its total calories are from the dressing alone–*quite a lot if you ask me.*

## Salads

Next, we have salads. The biggest mistake made with salads, aside from adding ladles worth of dressing to them, comes from what I like to call, *"salad extras,"* like:

- Avocado
- Beans
- Cheese
- Croutons
- Fruit and Dried Fruit
- Nuts and Seeds

**The reason salads are deemed a healthy staple is because they contain lots of nutrient-dense vegetables and they're low in calories–*supposedly.***

---

[18] The 99's Garden Salad and Honey Mustard Dressing calorie and macro totals were taken from the nutritional menu given on their website.

Let's take a look at two salads below. Although similar, the macro profiles of these two salads are much different. **Salad (1) contains only 170 calories, whereas Salad (2) has _700 more_ and over _10 times the amount of fat!_**

### Salad (1)

### Salad (2)

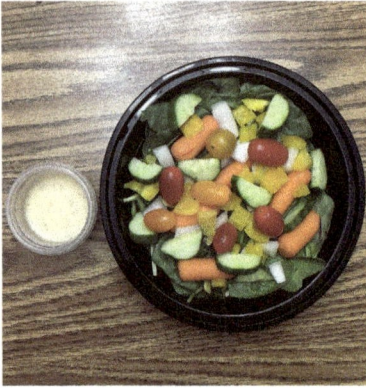
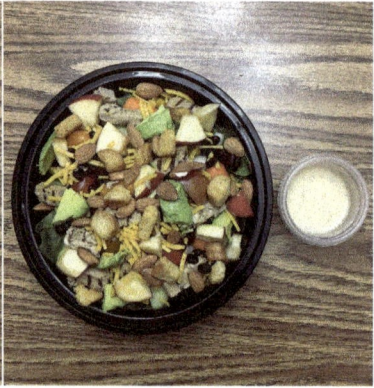

- **Calories:** 170
- **Carbs:** 29 g
- **Protein:** 5 g
- **Fat:** 4 g

- **Calories:** 870
- **Carbs:** 73 g
- **Protein:** 38 g
- **Fat:** 47 g

Why is this? Because Salad (2) has all the same vegetables as does Salad (1); but it also has a lot of salad extras:

- Almonds
- Apple Slices
- Avocado
- Beyond Meat Chicken Strips
- Black Beans
- Croutons

- Daiya Cheese

And it's paired with a traditional Italian dressing versus the light Italian dressing with Salad (1).

Does this mean, though, that you shouldn't eat Salad (2) and never add any salad extras to your salads? *Not at all!* **Avocado, beans, fruit, and nuts are very nutrient-dense foods; all of which I regularly add to my own salads. They're just calorically dense and you need to be aware of this, especially if you're eating a salad thinking it's the** *"lighter"* **option;** or because you're just trying to eat healthier overall. **Calories can add up quickly,** *even the healthy ones!*

**If you like loading your salad with a lot of extras, then I suggest using a light dressing option over a traditional one–preferably with 50 calories or less per serving.** Using light dressings, in general, will help reduce the total amount of calories you take in. Coconut and liquid aminos are two great low-calorie dressings for salads, as well, and are what I often use on my own salads and Buddha Bowls.

If you'd still prefer to use a traditional dressing, then by all means go for it. **Be mindful of how much you're using, add it into your calories, and you'll be good!**

## Nuts & Nut Butters

Has this ever been you?
- **Friend:** *"Did you have any protein with your breakfast this morning?"*
- **You:** *"Yeah, I had some peanut butter on my toast."*

If so, don't worry because there are many more alike. Nuts and nut butter are easily two of the most common foods mistaken for a good source of protein. **Yes, nuts do contain a decent amount of protein and they're very healthy for you. However, compared to the other macronutrients, their protein content isn't nearly as significant.**

For example, in a two-tablespoon serving of **Smucker's Natural Chunky Peanut Butter**, there are eight grams of protein; but also six grams of carbs, *16 grams of fat,* and 200 calories. In the same two-tablespoon serving of **MaraNatha's Crunchy Almond Butter,** there are seven grams of protein; but also six grams of carbs, another *16 grams of fat,* and 195 calories.

To compare these to a *lean* source of protein, one scoop (31 grams) of **PEScience's Peanut Butter Delight Vegan Protein Powder** contains 110 calories, **20 grams of protein,** four grams of carbs, and only one gram of fat.

To acquire that same 20 grams of protein through just Smucker's Chunky Peanut Butter, you'd have to consume 92 grams. **In those 92 grams worth of peanut butter, there are 20 grams of protein; but also 17 grams of carbs, *and 54 grams of fat! A whopping 600 calories worth of peanut butter just to get 20 grams of protein!***

Just because something has protein, doesn't mean it's a *lean* source of protein. **Lean protein sources have at least *two to three times more protein* than both their carbs and fat (not including fiber).**[19]

---

[19] See the "Best Nutrient-Dense Plant-Protein" list, page 97.

## Cooked vs. Uncooked Calories

The most common mistake I see for those new to calorie counting is not knowing the nutrient difference between cooked and uncooked food. This is a problem because **when food is cooked, the serving size will typically yield a different macro profile due to the cooking process.** A great example of this is quinoa.

When quinoa is dry and uncooked, the serving size listed has fewer calories per gram than when cooked because the grain retains the water that it's cooked in. Meaning, it'll weigh more once cooked after it's absorbed the water.

Easy Quinoa by Nature's Earthly Choice (¼ Cup Dry) (43 g)
- **Dry:** 170 kcals, 2.5 g fat, 24 g carbs, 7 g protein
- **Cooked:** 85 kcals, 1.5 g fat, 12 g carbs, 3.5 g protein

**In 43 grams of cooked Easy Quinoa by Nature's Earthly Choice, there are only half the number of calories and macros than when it's dry and uncooked–***a huge difference!*

A reverse example of this is meat and seafood. When you buy meat and seafood (although I suggest that you don't), the label on the package gives the uncooked nutritional data based on the raw weight. Raw meat and seafood contain a lot of water. While cooking, much of this water evaporates, causing it to become lighter once cooked.

For example, four ounces of raw shrimp has fewer calories than does four ounces cooked, as that four ounces raw won't weigh four ounces when cooked–*it'll weigh less.* This means that the macro profile for four ounces of cooked shrimp came from a heavier raw weight.

Shrimp (4 oz.) (113 g) [1]
- **Raw:** 75 kcals, 1 g fat, 1 g carbs, 15 g protein
- **Cooked:** 130 kcals, 2 g fat, 2 g carbs, 26 g protein

As you can see, there are 55 more calories in four ounces of cooked shrimp per the same weight than when raw, as well as a gram more of both carbs and fat, and 11 more grams of protein. **Knowing these differences is necessary so that you can log your food in its correct state and ensure the accuracy of your counting.**

## Underestimating Portion Sizes

**Although** *what* **you're eating is important,** *how much* **you're eating matters most!** *Calories in versus calories burned.* And this will make a big difference if you're counting but underestimating portion sizes.

Using nuts as an example again, when asked how many nuts someone ate for a snack, the most common response I hear is, *"a handful or two."* But how much exactly is a *"handful?"* In the picture on the next page taken from my Instagram **(@bobbyphysique),** I'm holding a *"handful"* of cashews in each hand.

However, these are two very different handfuls, as one weighs precisely one ounce (28 grams), and the other is twice the size at two ounces (56 grams). In terms of volume, it doesn't look like much of a difference. But in terms of calories and macros, *the difference is enormous!*

**The handful on the left has only 160 calories and 13 grams of fat, but the handful on the right has** *320 calories and 26 grams of fat!* So, yes, maybe you did only have one or two *"handfuls"* of nuts for your mid-afternoon snack, *but how many calories and macros did you take in?* That's the real question.

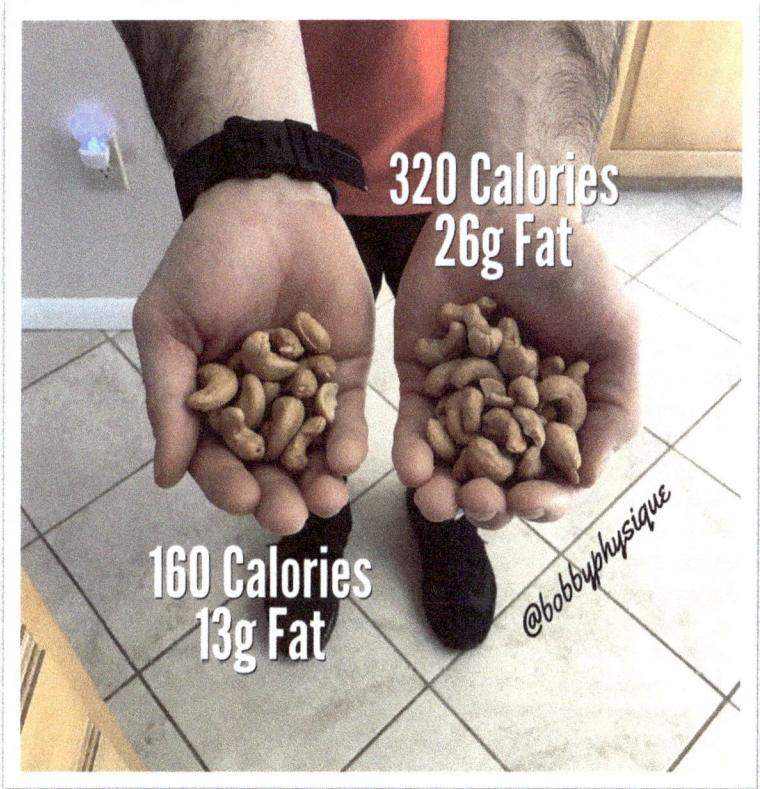

320 Calories
26g Fat

160 Calories
13g Fat

@bobbyphysique

**This is why it's helpful to measure or weigh the portions of your food.** If you've never counted your calories before but go right to guessing your portion sizes, you'll likely underestimate what you're consuming. This could lead to many untracked calories and quickly push you over your daily limit. **If you're not seeing results even though you've been consistently eating** *"better,"* **it's because you're still overeating.**

Before you can become a master calorie counter and intuitive eater, you first need to learn portion sizes. This can be done over time through daily calorie counting.

## Chapter Conclusion

If you're eating *"healthy,"* but your results are stagnant or going in the opposite direction, chances are one or all of these common food mistakes are to blame.

Remember, **what will ultimately determine the changes in your physique is your caloric intake and output.** So, even if you:

- Drink caloric drinks.
- Use oil when you cook.
- Use regular dressings.
- Add salad extras to your salads.
- Eat nuts and nut butter.
- All of the above.

**You can still lose weight, as long as you're eating less than you're burning.** It's just important to be aware that all of these things are calorically dense. **Count your calories accurately and see what a difference it'll make!**

# Restaurants, Fast Food & Alcohol

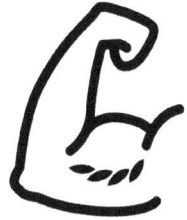

It's Wednesday, it's nearing midday, and you're sitting at your desk at work. Your stomach is rumbling, as you haven't eaten anything since breakfast five hours earlier and you're waiting for the clock to strike noon to go on break.

Finally, the last few seconds tick by, and it's time. You quickly rush from your desk to the break room, rip open the fridge only to realize that you forgot to pack your lunch this morning because Sparky pooped on the rug and you had to clean it up before heading out the door. Now, what do you do?

*To Chipotle it is!*

But wait a minute.

Didn't you just start your *"diet"* on Monday? *You can't be eating Chipotle!* *Sulks head and slowly walks back to desk*

Sound familiar? Maybe not the part about Sparky pooping on the rug (or that, too), but the part about not eating at restaurants or fast food joints because you're *"dieting,"* and food from those places is now somehow forbidden?

It does to me, as it's something I hear new clients tell me often. Yes, I advise against eating at places like Burger King, McDonald's, Taco Bell, etc., because the food is basically toxic waste. But, to reach (and maintain) your physique goals, *what* **you eat is not as important as is** *how much* **you eat of it;** although, don't get me wrong, what you eat is *very* important for your overall health and longevity (80|20 Rule).

## Nutrition Information

Nowadays, you can find almost anything on the internet (which isn't always a good thing lol), including the nutritional information for many restaurants. Most chain restaurants like Chipotle, Olive Garden, and even McDonald's have their nutrition facts right on their website. Some also have custom nutritional calculators based on their specific menu; **Chipotle** is one of them!

### My Suggestion

If you're counting your calories, visit the website of the restaurant you're dining at and see if their nutritional info is available. If it is, add in your meal based on the facts provided before you eat it, and make sure that it stays within your goals. Even if you're not counting, I still recommend checking the website for the calories and macros to help with intuitively eating throughout the rest of the day.

If a restaurant doesn't provide its nutritional info (which is typical for most family-owned restaurants), that's okay, too! There are many different ways to control the caloric intake of your meal, and the following restaurant tips will teach you how to do just that.

# General Restaurant Tips

Drinks

Water! **Water!** *Water!*

As your meal will likely have a lot of calories, it's best not to drink them, too. Whether dining out or eating at home, I always stick to just water. If you're not a fan of plain water, then get water with lemon or lime in it to add some flavor.

If you'd still prefer to have a flavored drink like juice or soda, then go with the diet or unsweetened version; as juice and soda are calorically dense. The same goes for alcoholic beverages. Margaritas and mixed drinks tend to be the highest in calories. The standard 32-ounce frozen margarita served at most restaurants is upwards of 600 calories *or more!*

### My Suggestion

If you're having a margarita, get it on the rocks rather than frozen; as the ice will significantly reduce the amount of liquid and, therefore, calories. For mixed drinks (made with beer, juice, or soda), ask for them to be made with a light alternative like club soda or light beer. Regardless, **always limit yourself to one small glass at a time and match each glass with a glass of water.** This goes for all drinks–beer, juice, margaritas, mixed drinks, wine, and soda alike.

## Oil & Butter

The main priority of restaurants is taste, as the taste of their food directly reflects on their success. Therefore, most restaurants cook using lots of oil or butter because they add flavor to the dish. But as we just learned, cooking with oil and butter is one of the most common food mistakes; as both are calorically dense and add a ton of hidden calories.

If on the menu, you see a dish described as *"breaded," "roasted," "fried," or "stir-fried,"* then this indicates that it was prepared using oil or butter.

### My Suggestion

Ask for your meal to be prepared without oil or butter and to be **steamed with water** instead. This will significantly decrease the total amount of calories of the dish. If you'd rather have it prepared as is, that's perfectly okay. If I'm not dieting for fat loss, I usually only ask to have my veggies steamed, as that's how I prefer them. Just know though that your fat intake for the day will be high and you should consume far less during the rest of your meals.

Oil and butter are also commonly served on their own as a complement to bread. You'll see this a lot at Italian restaurants.

### My Suggestion

Ask for a side of marinara sauce or vinegar, instead, or simply eat the bread plain (what I do myself).

Butter also isn't vegan and so if you're vegan, then this is something you'll definitely want to avoid.

## Dressings & Sauces

- Ask for the light option.
- Ask for it on the side.

If there aren't any light dressings or sauces available, then go with your favorite normal one, but always ask for it on the side. One too many times I've put faith in my server to lightly coat my salad, and one too many times I've been served a bowl of dressing with my salad on top (*face in palm*).

**Having your dressings and sauces served on the side allows you full control over how much is used, ultimately reducing your consumption of unnecessary calories.**

## Fasting

Let's put things into perspective. It's Saturday, and you're meeting friends tonight for dinner. Your restaurant of choice is The Cheesecake Factory (one of my personal favorites). If you've ever been to The Cheesecake Factory, then you know that their meals, let alone their 1,500-plus-calorie pieces of cheesecake, are calorically dense. Add in an appetizer, complimentary bread, and any caloric drinks; and, before you know it, your calories for that meal could easily be upwards of 5,000 or more! This isn't even counting all the other food you probably already ate that day, too.

**This is where fasting can be beneficial.**

If you know you'll be eating out at night, then eat light but filling meals consisting of lean protein, veggies, and complex carbs, during the day. **Beans, lentils, and potatoes are great voluminous carb choices; while Seitan, TVP, lean mock meats, and protein powder are great lean protein ones.** This, combined with a sufficient intake of water, will keep you full leading up to dinner; but will also leave plenty of calories reserved for your calorically dense meal still to come.

**Then, while at the restaurant, think balance.** For example, most desserts are calorically dense and very high in sugar and fat. If you want to have dessert, for your main course have something lighter and also consisting of lean protein and veggies.

You might also want to share an appetizer (and your dessert, too) and eat only one or two pieces of complimentary bread instead of five or six. Drink lots of water throughout the meal and *there you go!* You just enjoyed dinner out with friends without having to trash your diet.

*Great job!*

**Following this large meal is the ideal time to fast with an increased water intake for 12-16 hours or more to allow your body the time it needs to digest and reset.** Once this time has passed, slowly resume eating as usual, preferably by starting with a small meal of lean protein and veggies to balance out your nutrients.

If, however, you're going to a restaurant but don't plan on having a large meal, then don't worry about fasting. Follow the first three general restaurant tips, eat intuitively, count your calories if possible (and if you're currently counting), relax, and *enjoy yourself!*

## Alcohol

Alcohol is perfectly okay to consume (and is sometimes even healthy), as long as it's in moderation:

- One drink* per day for women.
- Up to two drinks* per day for men.

*A drink is defined as one 5-ounce glass of wine, 12-ounce beer, or a 1-ounce shot of hard liquor.* [25]

If consumed in excess, however, alcohol can have many adverse effects on your body, performance, and results; such as:

- Weight gain
- The loss of fluids and electrolytes from its diuretic effect
- Increased sweating and lactic acid
- Dehydration
- Decreased testosterone
- Elevated cortisol levels
- Muscle loss and the prevention of muscle protein synthesis
- Impaired reaction time, balance, and hand-eye coordination

This is why **alcohol should never be consumed before or during exercise and competition.** Doing so will significantly hurt your performance and could lead to serious injury.

Furthermore, **alcohol is calorically dense (seven calories per gram) and quickly leads to weight gain when overeating.** However, because alcohol is toxic and can't be stored within the body, your body digests it first and slows the digestion of other nutrients until burned. This means that **the weight you gain from too much drinking will come from everything else you've eaten, and not from the alcohol itself.** Again, however, this only happens when, overall, you're consuming more than you're burning. [7]

## Positive Effects
**Moderate red wine consumption has been shown to increase healthy cholesterol and reduce the risk of vascular disease.** However, these positive benefits are likely to be seen only in people age 45 and older. [28]

Alcohol also helps people relax socially; which makes for a better time when going out. Nevertheless, overconsumption is still harmful to overall fitness; but so is eating too much and overtraining. Thus, the saying goes, *"everything in moderation."* **If you like alcohol, then consume it moderately; avoid consumption around exercise and competition, and you'll be good.**

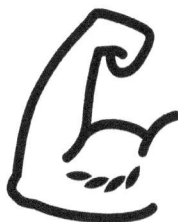

# Supplements

Before we get started, I'm going to answer one of the most common nutritional questions, *"are supplements necessary to achieving your health and fitness goals (fat burners, pre-workout, testosterone boosters, vitamins, etc.)?"*

The short answer? **No.** The long answer? ***HELL NO!***

Can supplements be helpful? Some of them, yes, like protein powder, BCAAs, and specific vitamins and minerals when needed. **But fat burners, testosterone boosters, and all the *"magic pills"* claiming they'll *"eat the fat"* or help you *"lose 10 pounds in 10 days"* are *100% unnecessary!***

They're garbage, and if you've ever noticed the disclaimers on them, they all say, *"results not guaranteed"* and *"must be taken in combination with proper diet and exercise."* Because, ultimately, **that's all that's necessary–*proper diet and exercise,* combined with a little commitment, consistency, and accountability.**

## The Science Behind Fat Burners

Fat burners (predominantly the caffeine within them) stimulate our *"fight-or-flight"* hormones (epinephrine and norepinephrine). These hormones then stimulate the release of fatty acids into the bloodstream for energy. They also suppress appetite and gastric function. [7]

It's for these reasons one would think that by just taking a fat burner, it should burn their fat. However, **without exercise, the fatty acids released into the bloodstream won't be used. If there isn't any increased muscle activity that needs the energy, they simply get recycled back to fat storage.** This is why fat burners *"must be taken in combination with proper diet and exercise."* If they're not, then you won't experience the benefits of your *"fight-or-flight"* hormones being released. [7]

These hormones can also be stimulated by other things, as well—exercise and stress two of the most common. Therefore, just by working out and challenging your muscles, your fat-burning hormones are released naturally, and you burn fat without having to exercise your wallet too. [7]

Regarding caffeine, specifically, it's been shown to boost performance. [7] But again, you can consume caffeine when needed naturally through coffee, various teas, or caffeinated plant-based energy bars like **BTC Bars** (use code *"BobbyPhysique20"* for 20% off any order).

So, if at burners aren't really necessary, then why do so many people buy them?

Unfortunately, because many people would prefer the *"quick fix"* that they're sold on TV and the internet, rather than putting in the work necessary to build their dream physique. They want results *fast,* and they want them *now!* But the fact is, *the quicker the fix, the faster the relapse.* **If you want** *results that last,* **then you need to dedicate the time and effort to produce them...Period!**

## Recommended Supplements

With all of that said, although supplements aren't necessary, and you can obtain everything you need (vitamins, minerals, fiber, and protein) through a plant-based diet; there are still some supplements that I take myself and that I recommend if they help *"supplement"* your nutrition.

## Vitamin $B_{12}$ (Debunking the Myth)

As a vegan, the first supplement that I always recommend to fellow plant-based eaters is vitamin $B_{12}$ because it's essential for DNA and red blood cell production. It also prevents anemia, nerve damage, neurocognitive changes, and paralysis, all of which are very serious conditions.

Vitamin $B_{12}$ comes from bacteria found in dirt and soil. The reason it's easily obtained through meat and animal products is that:
1.  The food the animals eat is covered with this dirt and soil.
2.  It's also lined in their guts. [28]

And so, when these animals and their by-products are consumed, their $B_{12}$ is passed onto us.

**Humans also produce vitamin $B_{12}$ within the gut, however, only in the colon.** This means that we're unable to absorb what we make, as $B_{12}$ is only absorbed in the small intestine which is upstream of the colon. This wasn't a problem for prehistoric populations because, similar to the farm animals of today, the plant foods they ate were covered in dirt and soil filled with $B_{12}$. However, because of the thorough washing, cleaning, and cooking process that we put our food through now, we reduce the $B_{12}$ content of the plant foods we eat. [28]

So, although a plant-based diet is full of many other vitamins and minerals, it's typically low in vitamin $B_{12}$. This puts vegans and vegetarians at risk for $B_{12}$ deficiency, which is why many anti-vegans and paleo-enthusiasts say that you should eat meat.

But don't let all of that scare (or fool) you because vitamin B$_{12}$ deficiency can be easily prevented. And, in fact, **one in six meat eaters is actually B$_{12}$ deficient themselves.** [28]

Vitamin B$_{12}$ can be found in many fortified foods such as certain cereals, plant milk, soymilk, and nutritional yeast. Many energy drinks also have over 100% of the recommended daily dose, as well. However, the easiest and most reliable way to ensure adequate intake is through an oral supplement.

For the average adult, it's recommended to take **350 micrograms (mcg) per day** or **2,500 per week.** [28] Personally, I take just one 2,500 microgram dose each week for convenience, but either way works.

## Vitamin D$_3$

The only other vitamin supplement that I take, aside from Vitamin B$_{12}$, is Vitamin D$_3$, as it's necessary for proper calcium absorption and bone growth. However, I only supplement with it during the winter months when my sun exposure is limited; and I'm rarely consistent with it.

If you live in a colder region where your sun exposure is minimal, then I suggest getting your levels checked and supplementing if yours are low. It's common for women from the northeastern states of America to be Vitamin D$_3$ deficient. [7] **But as long as you get at least 30 minutes of sun each day, your D$_3$ levels will be perfectly fine!**

Be aware, however, that **most Vitamin D$_3$ supplements are *not* vegan, as they're often derived from an animal source like sheep's wool.** [38] So, if you're vegan and are looking for a good D$_3$ supplement, **Garden of Life** makes a great vegan one.

## Protein Powder

Protein powder isn't necessary, and you can build muscle and thrive by solely eating plant foods and enough calories of them. However, I like to supplement with a scoop of protein powder almost every day (but mainly on my workout days), which ensures that I'm getting plenty of protein and essential amino acids exactly when I need them most.

Most vegan protein powders are made from either a pea protein, brown rice protein, or a blend of both. I've also seen some made from chia seed, hemp seed, pumpkin seed, sunflower seed, and even watermelon seed, as well.

My favorite vegan protein powders, all of which contain 18-20 grams of protein or more per serving, are:
- **PEScience Vegan Select Series**
- **Sunwarrior Warrior Blend**
- **Vivo Life Perform**
- **Orgain Organic Plant-Based Protein**
- **Garden of Life Raw Organic Protein**

## BCAAs

**Branched-chain amino acids (BCAAs)** *consist of the three essential amino acids leucine, isoleucine, and valine. Unlike the other six essential amino acids, BCAAs are mostly metabolized in the skeletal muscle rather than the liver. Because of this, their primary function is **muscle protein synthesis:** the process of building muscle, which not only builds it but also protects against its breakdown and damage.* [7]

Protein breakdown and synthesis continually happen throughout the body and increase during exercise. Therefore, it's necessary to consume an adequate amount of BCAAs every day, especially during and around training to properly promote these functions. Doing so will help maximize your workouts, reduce muscle loss (very important when dieting for fat loss), delay fatigue, and help with recovery. This also goes for vegans, vegetarians, and meat eaters alike.

**When supplementing, aim for a 2:1:1 or 3:1:1 ratio of leucine to valine to isoleucine.** [7]

However, be aware that, **unless they're labeled vegan, most BCAA supplements are made from duck feathers, pig fur, and even human hair. Yes, you read that right–h***uman hair!* **I'm not kidding!** Thus, the best BCAAs to buy are plant-based and certified vegan. The only vegan ones I've tried so far are **Vivo Life's Sustain BCAAs,** and they're delicious!

**When supplementing, I've had the best results taking BCAAs during my workouts; but they may also be taken immediately before or after exercise.** However, if you'd rather not spend the extra money for a separate BCAA pill or powder, then don't worry. Most protein powders are fortified with a complete amino acid profile, including BCAAs and all other essential and nonessential aminos. So, by just supplementing with a scoop of protein every day, you'll get everything you need, and more. **But, again, you can also obtain all of your essential aminos by consuming plant-based foods and enough calories of them.**

## Iron

Although you can easily consume plenty of iron on a plant-based diet, the downside is that plant sources aren't as bioavailable as are meat sources; which means that it's harder for the body to absorb the iron from plant foods.

Therefore, because women lose a lot of iron during their monthly period, I recommend supplementing if you're a vegan or vegetarian woman. **A** low-level dose of 18-20 milligrams (mg) per day in combination with vitamin C to aid with proper absorption is plenty. I recommend **Iron Plus C by Vital Nutrients.**

If you'd prefer not to supplement, then **the best natural sources of iron are:**
- **Legumes:** Lentils, soybeans, tofu, tempeh, lima beans, black beans, chickpeas
- **Grains:** Quinoa, fortified cereals, brown rice, oatmeal
- **Nuts & Seeds:** Pumpkin seeds, squash seeds, pine nuts, pistachios, sunflower seeds, cashews, un-hulled sesame seeds
- **Vegetables:** Tomato sauce, Swiss chard, collard greens
- **Other:** Blackstrap molasses, prune juice

## All the Rest
**Unless you have a specific deficiency, there's no need to supplement with any other vitamins or minerals.**

**For herbs and spices,** there are a few that I regularly use for their positive benefits. These include:
- **Apple Cider Vinegar:** Aids digestion and strengthens immune system.
- **Cinnamon:** Loaded with antioxidants, is anti-inflammatory, and lowers blood sugar.
- **Black Pepper:** Aids digestion and enhances **bioavailability** *(a measure of the absorption of nutrients by the body).*
- **Garlic:** Strengthens immune system.
- **Ginger:** Anti-inflammatory.
- **Maca Root Powder:** Supports healthy sexual function and libido, increases energy and endurance, and reduces anxiety and stress.

- **Turmeric:** Anti-inflammatory and strengthens immune system.

Other than that, I get all of my necessary nutrients through the foods I eat; *and so can you!* **As long as the majority of what you consume is plant-based (like fruit, vegetables, whole grains, beans, legumes, nuts, seeds, tofu, tempeh, seitan, and other lean protein sources), then you'll receive everything you need *and more!***

# Part 6

# Intuitive Eating

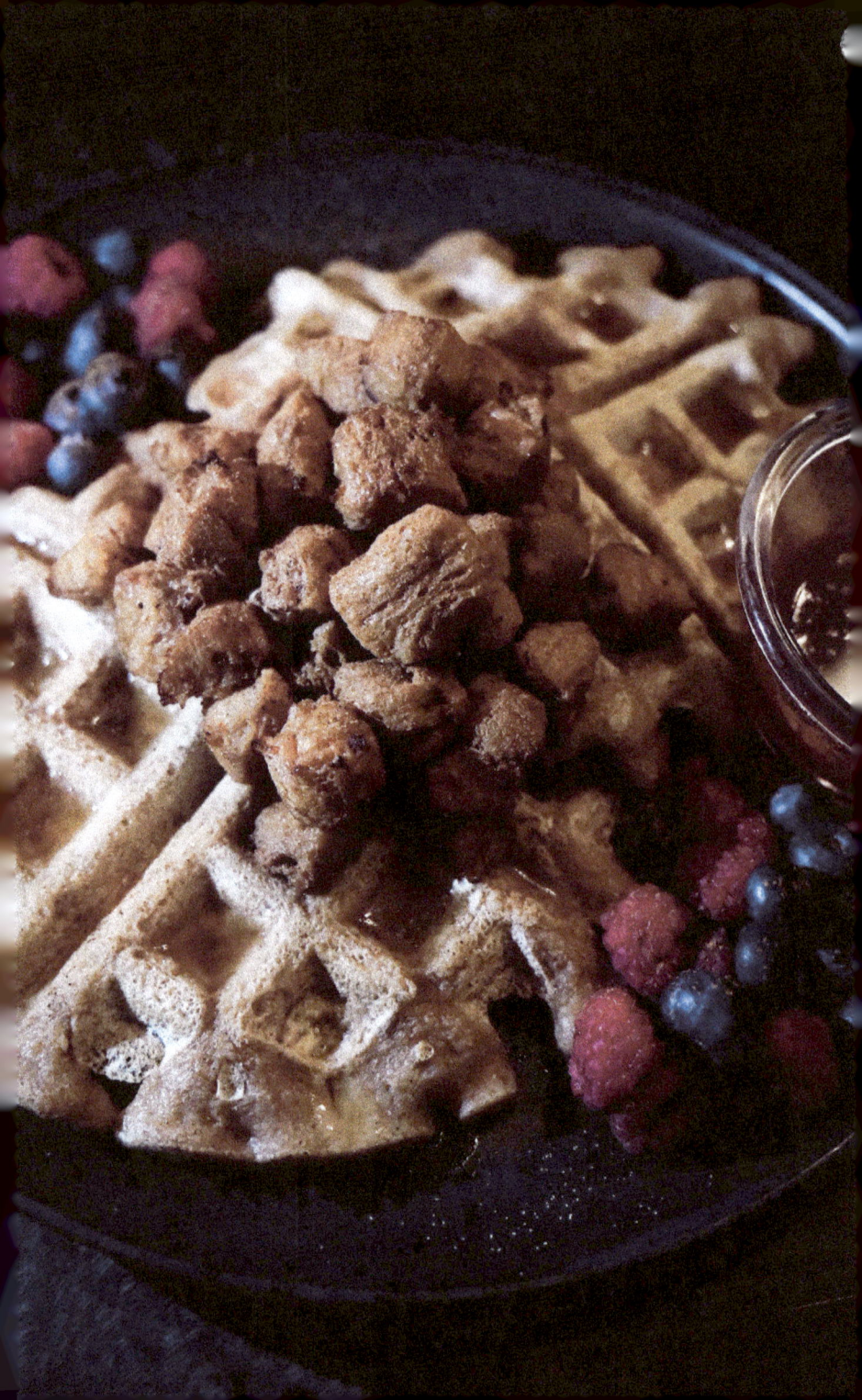

**6.1**

# What is Intuitive Eating?

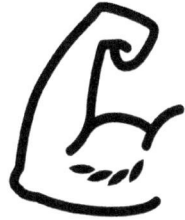

The ability to eat intuitively is a natural skill that all of us are born with. Our bodies know when we're hungry, and they know when we've had enough. In primal times, if you were too skinny and never ate enough or were too heavy and always overate, you'd be at risk for survival.

This is why our bodies naturally regulate themselves and our eating so that we maintain an optimal level of **homeostasis:** *a balance of energy in versus energy burned.* [7] You might ask then, if this is the case, *why are so many people today overweight?*

That answer is revealed in our market and society that's saturated with calorically dense, nutrient-stripped, high-fat, processed, and sugary foods. Not only do these foods disrupt our bodies' hormones and cause us to gain weight and fall ill; but they also make us want to eat more, as they're engineered to do.

Our society, as are the societies of all industrialized countries, is always on the go. We're constantly busy and going from one thing to the next. This often causes us to eat too quickly and mindlessly; as we're often distracted while eating by our coworkers, cellphone, commute, kids, TV, etc.

**To feel full, it takes a solid 15-20 minutes for your body to process that feeling after you're already at the point of *being* full.** Thus, when we eat too fast without thinking, we aren't tuned into our hunger and fullness cues, and we tend to overeat.

These hunger and fullness cues are also tuned out because of our environment and societal norms:
- Eat what you want, when you want, wherever you are.
- Always finish your plate, don't waste food.
- It's a certain time–*eat.*
- It's a certain event–*eat.*
- You're emotional–*eat.*
- You're bored–*go eat.*
- You're reminded of food (which is almost constantly)–*chow down and eat!* [7]

Obesity wasn't an issue during prehistoric times because genetically modified processed foods weren't a thing yet, nor was industrial society. Humans only ate natural foods that were grown from the ground or raised in the wild, ones that our have been designed to process. [7]

This is why calorie counting in today's world is extremely useful because it teaches you what's going in and out of your body. **The more time you devote to counting, the more knowledgeable you'll become about the macro profiles of the food you regularly eat. This base knowledge will then allow you to eat intuitively, as you'll be able to make better-informed decisions while still building in those empty calories you love.**

Now, what is intuitive eating exactly?

**Intuitive eating is:**
- Always being in tune with your body's hunger and fullness cues, wants, and needs.

- Being mindful and eating when hungry and stopping when satiated.
- For the majority of the time, making food choices based on nutrient density, quality, and if the food is believed to be satisfying.
- Choosing whether or not to indulge in cravings and *not letting them choose you!* [7]

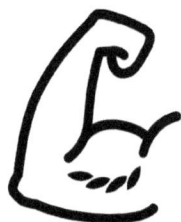

# How to Eat Intuitively

## 1. Slow Down

**Eating intuitively means being mindful and aware of what you're eating** *(and doing).* Instead of eating while watching TV, scrolling mindlessly through Instagram, or in the car while rushing to your next appointment; put the distractions aside and devote mealtimes to yourself.

**The best ways to practice slowing down while eating are to:**
- Schedule mealtimes.
- Time yourself while eating.
- Count your chews with each bite.

### Scheduling
If you're always busy and struggling with irregular eating habits, schedule dedicated mealtimes without distractions. Just like your workouts, **these mealtimes are to be treated like business meetings that are** *not* **optional;** except these meetings are for yourself and your health, which is, above all, *the most important thing* in your life. **If you're not in good health,** *nothing else matters!*

### Timing
During your mealtimes, if eating too fast is an issue for you, time yourself while eating. **Ideally, each meal should take you at least 15 minutes**

**to finish.** This will give your body the proper time it needs to start digesting your food and determine whether it's satiated or not.

Once finished, if necessary, time yourself again by waiting for at least another 15 minutes. If after 15 minutes has passed from the time you finished eating and you're still hungry, then go ahead and eat a little more. Again, *going slowly.*

### Chewing
**While eating, to best help yourself slow down, every time you put food in your mouth, chew it at least 20-30 times before swallowing.** Focus on the flavor. Feel the texture. Really savor your food and enjoy each bite.

## 2. Practice Noticing Your Cues
Once you've mastered eating slowly, the next step is to practice noticing your cues *before* you start eating and *after* you're finished.

**When you feel hungry,** before running to the fridge or cabinet, stop and think about what else your body's feeling.
- Is my stomach growling? Does it feel empty?
- Am I lightheaded?
- What have I already eaten today?
- Have I eaten enough veggies? Starchy carbs? Fiber? Lean protein?
- Have I drunk enough water?
- Did I already consume a lot of calories, processed foods, sugar, and fat?
- Have I not eaten enough yet?

Once you've decided that you're actually hungry and that you're going to have a meal, ask yourself similar questions once you've finished eating that meal.

- Do I feel full? Overtly stuffed? Extra heavy?
- Is my stomach upset because I ate too much?
- Am I simply satisfied because I've have had enough?

**Intuitive eating is *balanced* eating.** If you already had a large meal (or meals) earlier that day or the day before, for your next one or two, eat a little less and focus on consuming what your body needs. If your previous meal was very high in carbs and fat, then your next should consist of more lean protein and veggies; or vice versa, if you're low on carbs and fat, then have some more.

**Again, counting calories helps with becoming more aware of the calories and macros you're consuming, as you'll be able to clearly see what you've already eaten and what more you need.**

## 3. Use the Hunger & Fullness Scale

Another helpful way to notice your cues is by using the Hunger & Fullness Scale. To do this, think of your hunger and fullness on scale from 1-10:

- 1 being *"Ravenous."*
- 10 being *"Overstuffed."*

### Hunger & Fullness Scale

| 1 | 2 | 3 | 4 | 5 |
|---|---|---|---|---|
| Ravenous | Very Hungry | Hungry | Slightly Hungry | Neutral |

| 6 | 7 | 8 | 9 | 10 |
|---|---|---|---|---|
| Satisfied | Slightly Full | Full | Very Full | Overstuffed |

When listening to your cues, on this scale you should start eating around 2-3 (20-30% hungry) and stop eating around 7-8 (70-80% full). [7] Doing this will ensure that you stay *ahead* of your hunger, so that when you sit down to eat, you're not ready to eat through the fridge. It'll also ensure that you stop before getting overstuffed, allowing your body the chance to process the food you've eaten and register that it's full.

## 4. Journal

If you struggle with binging and emotional eating, then take the time to journal your behaviors around these eating episodes.

> "*Research shows that while our behaviors may seem 'spur-of-the-moment' when it comes to overeating, the groundwork is laid several hours in advance by our daily rituals, habits, mindset, and automatic thinking. **Overeating is simply the last link in a long chain. If you can break the first link, you have a much better chance of never getting to the last.**" [7]*

Every time you have an overeating episode, ask yourself the following questions and record your responses in a **behavior-awareness journal:**

1.  **In the 1-2 hours beforehand:**
    - What were you doing?
    - What were you thinking?
    - What were you feeling, emotionally?
    - What were you feeling, physically?
    - Where were you?
    - What time was it?
    - Who was with you?
2.  **Immediately beforehand:**
    - What were you doing?

- What were you thinking?
- What were you feeling, emotionally?
- What were you feeling, physically?
- Where were you?
- Who was with you?

3. **In the middle of it:**

   *The same questions as number two, plus:

   - What were you choosing to consume?
   - Why were you choosing these particular foods?

4. **Afterwards:**

   *The same questions as number two. [6]

**The goal of journaling is to build awareness of what these eating episodes have in common.** Maybe it's a time of day, or a situation, a type of food, another person (or being alone), a certain feeling–or all of these. It can also be used for slowing down and noticing your cues. [7]

**For slowing down,** use a **meal-duration journal** during meals and record:

- The time you start eating.
- What you're eating.
- The time you stop. [6]

**For noticing your cues,** use a **food-feelings journal** during meals and record:

- The time of day each meal is eaten.
- What you're eating.
- What you're feeling (emotionally and physically) before eating.
- What you're doing and thinking while eating.
- Any physical sensations that the food causes during eating and after you're finished. [6]

**Describe in as much detail as possible of what you remember experiencing at each stage, and then go back and review. This helps build an understanding of the process, which you can then use to disrupt unhealthy patterns.** [7]

For instance, if you habitually overeat in your kitchen at 6 p.m. when stressed; then figure out strategies to deal with a stressful dinner hour before it happens, as far in advance as possible. [7] For example, before dinner:

- Practice 10 minutes of meditation[20] or yoga.
- Go for a walk.
- Drink a satiating protein shake or munch on some fruit and veggies to help keep you full and away from the empty calories.

If you habitually think negative thoughts beforehand like, *"I'm a failure"* or *"eating this will make me feel better,"* then come up with ways to reframe these thoughts when they hit you. [7] For example:

- *"I'm not a failure, I've simply experienced a setback and can use this as an opportunity to learn."*
- *"This may satisfy me emotionally, but it might not help me physically."*

**Your mind is your most powerful tool. Simply changing your thought process can have a profound effect on the way you act, feel, and speak.[21] Stay positive and *relax*. You *can* and *will* achieve your goals!**

## Chapter Conclusion

Everyone is unique, which is why there's no one-size diet plan that fits

---

[20] See "Meditation," page 227.
[21] See "Mindset," page 7.

all. Developing the ability to eat intuitively in today's world is a skill that takes time and practice. Devote yourself to the learning process and to becoming more mindful when you eat. When you do so, your habits will slowly begin to change. And **when you build healthy habits, that's when you'll start to see *results that last!***

This isn't a diet. ***It's a LIFESTYLE!***

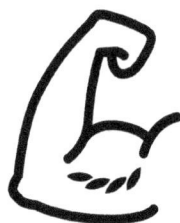

**6.3**

# Meditation

During the summer of 2018, I competed in my first physique competition. Afterward, I went through a period of post-show binging that morphed from just a couple weeks following my show, into over a couple months. During that time, *"intuitive eating"* wasn't a term in my vocabulary (although *"eating"* definitely was lol), as I was pushing *way beyond* fullness night after night.

After stepping off stage on June 15th through the end of September, I was consuming upwards of 5,000-6,000 calories almost every day (2,000-3,000 of which at night *after* eating dinner) and stuffing my face with pretty much anything and everything I could. I had lost control, and during that time, I vividly remember feeling like there was no end in sight.

I quickly became depressed. All I could think about was that I *"ruined"* the physique that I had worked so hard for months to achieve, within a matter of weeks. And I couldn't just snap my fingers and get it right back. This, in combination with other personal matters that I was dealing with at that time in my life, then led to more binging and emotional eating, more weight gain, and, ultimately, more depression and anxiety.

You know the *"snowball effect"* when a measly little snowball starts rolling down a mountain, and eventually, it grows and gets bigger until it turns into an avalanche? Yeah, that's what my life felt like then *times about 10!*

**Until I started meditating.**

I had been meditating sporadically during the earlier parts of 2018. But once I started practicing daily, I cannot tell you how much *better* I began to feel! Every day I made it a point to devote time to myself. Whether listening to an online meditation lesson, laying by the ocean, or sitting on my living room floor; 10-15 minutes each day was dedicated to meditation.

Slowly my mind stopped racing. My anxiety started to drift away. My depressive thoughts were staying in the past. Day-by-day my intuition came back. I could feel my mind connecting with my body again, and my hunger and fullness cues were no longer ignored.

**Meditating allowed me to become more mindful of how I was feeling and for *why* I was feeling that way.** More often than not, if I was feeling anxious or depressed (which I rarely do anymore), it's because I was overwhelmed and too focused on everything else other than the present moment. I would give situations–whether past, present, or future–more prominence than they deserved, and devote too much emotional energy into things beyond my control.

Now, however, whenever I feel anxious, depressed, or overwhelmed; instead of turning to food to temporarily ease the pain, I turn to meditation. I pause, take a deep breath, and bring myself back to here and now. I don't let my feelings get the best of me and, let me tell you, *what a difference it's made on so many levels!*

Meditation brought me back to being fully *me*–my happy and full-of-life self. And, if you follow the tips below, you can *take control* too!

## Steps to Meditating *(Taking Control)*

1. Find a quiet space
2. Sit (or lay) still
3. Close your eyes
4. Relax your shoulders
5. Breathe slowly
6. Breathe deeply
7. Center your mind
8. Let go

It doesn't matter where you are; as long as you have a place that's quiet where you can be alone, then that's a great place to be. My favorite places to meditate are the beach, the woods, my living room floor, and even my car. If you'd like to play soft deep-breathing, massage, or yoga music during this time or listen to an online meditation lesson, definitely feel free to do so.

Once I'm in my place, more often than not, I sit upright with my legs crossed and rest my hands on my knees. Sometimes I sit with my legs out straight, or I'll completely lay down flat on my back. Whatever feels most comfortable at the time and fits with where I'm at is what I do. No matter, I always ensure that my back is straight, and my palms are open and facing up.

Next, I close my eyes, relax my shoulders, and start taking slow, deep breaths. Of course, if I'm driving, I keep my eyes open (and I *highly* suggest you do too lol), but my breathing technique remains the same.

- I relax my shoulders.

- Use my diaphragm to fill my stomach with as much air as possible.
- Pause for a second at the top of each breath.
- Slowly let all the air out.
- Pause for a second at the bottom of each breath.
- Repeat.

Finally, I center my mind on my stomach and then *let go.* I let go of all thoughts and worries. I focus my attention on my breathing and let things flow. If unwanted thoughts come in (which they will, as your mind will always wander), I don't get mad or upset. I do my best to recognize them right away and then bring my attention back to center.

**The more accepting I am that thoughts will come and go as they please, the better I am with refocusing.**

If there's a lot on my mind, instead of letting go of my thoughts, I'll instead have an internal conversation with myself about them. If what I'm thinking about is a current life-conflict, then I'll seek to find what caused the problem **(starting with *my* contribution, first)** and what could remedy a solution. And, as always, I remind myself that *no obstacle is too big to overcome.* This positive self-talk allows me to approach the conflict better when it arises again and move towards a positive resolution.

**At the end of each meditation, I spend the last five minutes repeating positive mantras in my head.** This is my favorite part because, when I finish, I'm always in the best mood and truly feel like *no obstacle is too big to overcome!*

Practice these steps yourself. Devote time each day to be alone without distractions. I find the best time for me is first thing in the morning. I make sure to wake up early enough so that I have at least 10 minutes for meditation, as well as 10 minutes for stretching beforehand. Doing so allows me to start the day off right and ready to take on whatever comes my way! If it's a day where I'm planning a beach trip or a hike, then I'll save my meditation for when I go.

However, **no matter when you choose to meditate, you must *make it a habit!*** As with anything, **if you want to be successful with what you're doing, *then you must be consistent with doing it!***

Schedule time to meditate each day, *even if it's only 10-15 minutes.* Treat it as if it were a business meeting that's not optional, except this meeting is with yourself and for your health–*the most important thing in your life.* **Stay committed and watch just how much of a difference meditation will make!**

# Part 7

# Training

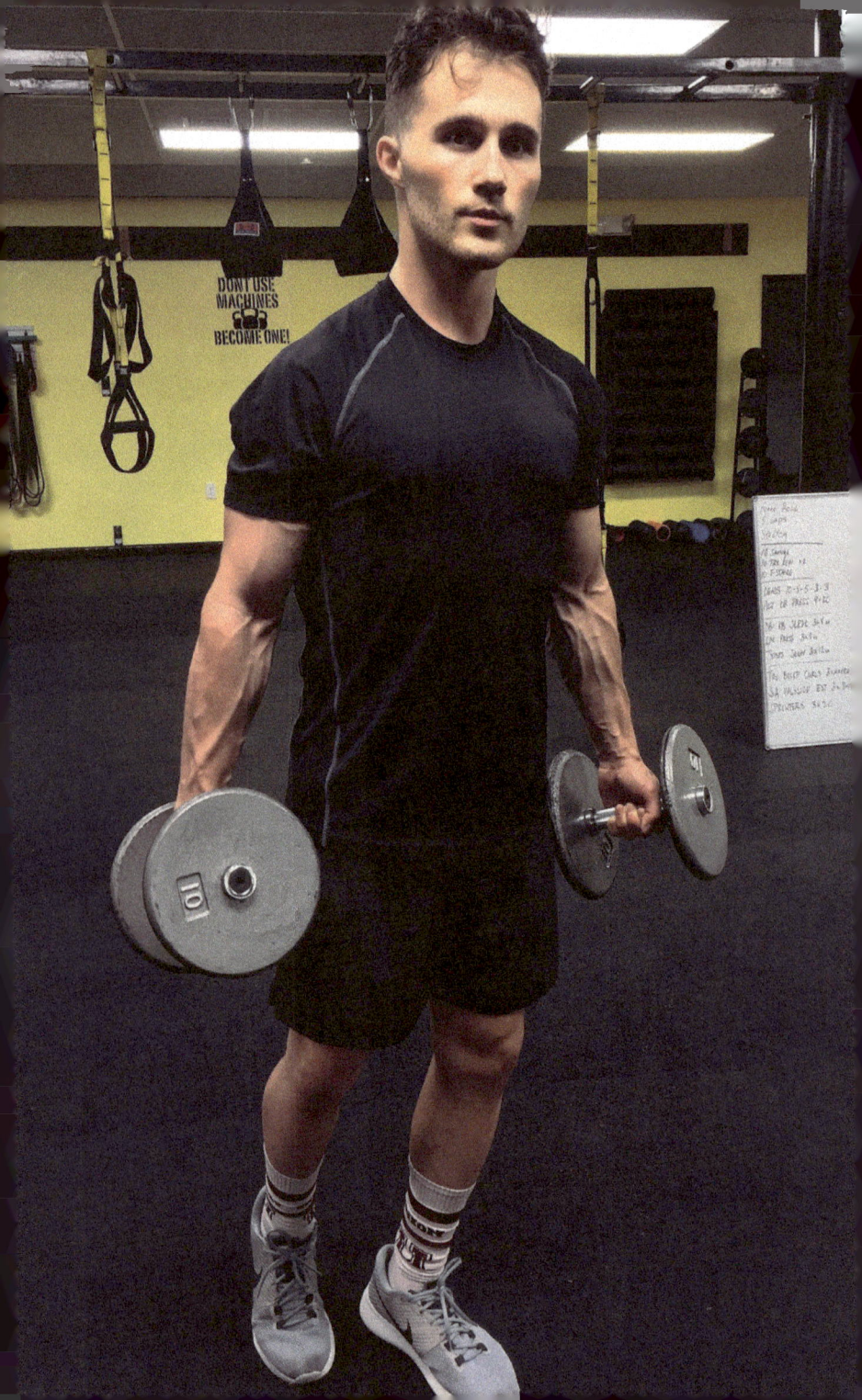

# The Importance of Diet
## *and Exercise*

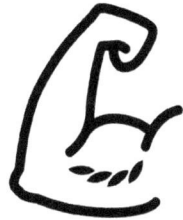

**Although diet should be your first priority, exercise is *equally* as important.** If your goal is to build a lean and *muscular* physique, then diet alone won't do it. You must exercise and more specifically, you must resistance train through either lifting weights, doing calisthenics (body-weight training), or both.

Ladies, *this means you too!* If you want that toned and curvy physique, then hitting the weights is what you should be doing; *not cardio!*

Low-intensity steady-state cardio **(LISS)** is **aerobic training** and it *conditions your slow-twitch (Type I) muscle fibers, which are large but thin.* Resistance training is **anaerobic training** and it *conditions your fast-twitch (Type II) muscle fibers, which are smaller but dense.* [28]

Consistently training your Type II muscle fibers builds muscle density, which is what you want. **The more muscle mass you have, the leaner you'll look at a higher BFP. You'll also be able to eat more in a resting state, as muscle requires more calories to sustain itself than fat does.**

Yes, cardio helps with heart conditioning and increasing caloric burn. But if you don't resistance train, and only do steady-state cardio when trying to lose weight, you'll just get skinny (or skinny fat).

To help illustrate this, look at Olympic sprinters versus long-distance runners. Whether male or female, the long-distance runners are thin with relatively little muscle mass, while the sprinters are toned and muscular.

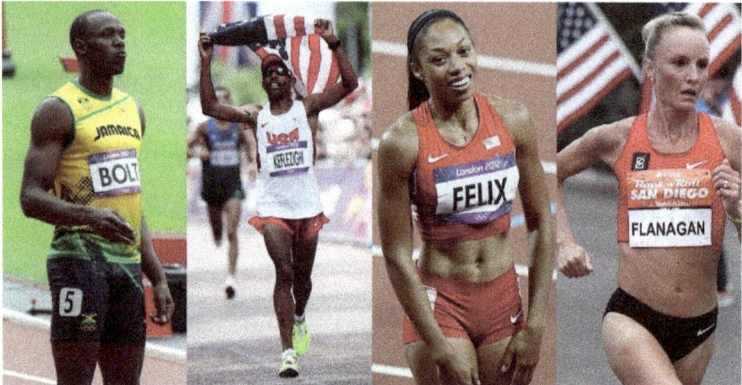

*In both pictures, the sprinters are on the left and the long-distance runners are on the right.*

This is because the long-distance runners mainly practice **LISS** and condition their Type I muscle fibers. Whereas the sprinters practice explosive resistance training and mainly condition their Type II's. **In other words, *stop doing hours on the elliptical!* It's only going to make you skinny and thin!**

Of course, if your goal is to run long distances (5k's, marathons, etc.), then long-distance running is what you should do. But otherwise, **if you want a lean and *muscular* physique, *then lift weights and lift heavy!***

**And ladies, don't worry about getting large and bulky like a man because *you physically can't.*** You don't produce enough testosterone naturally to do so. Lifting weights only makes you curvy and toned. Plus, because you produce much more estrogen than men, and estrogen greatly helps with recovery, you can work out more often and for longer durations because you'll recover faster! So again, **hit the weights and** *hit them hard!*

## Burn More, Eat More

Exercise is also essential because it allows you to eat more and still reach your goals.

For example, my daily BWMC based on my high activity level is roughly 3,000. Therefore, for me to lose one pound per week, I'd have to eat an average of 2,500 calories each day. However, if I weren't as active and I only had a daily maintenance level of 2,500, then I'd only be able to eat an average of 2,000 calories every day to lose the same pound each week. **Thus, the more you burn,** *the more you earn!*

## Additional Benefits

Aside from building and maintaining muscle and burning fat, exercise is also necessary for:
- Increasing strength and mobility.
- Preventing injury.
- Improving sports performance.
- Improving balance, posture, and stability.
- Improving brain function and memory.
- Elevating your mood.
- Alleviating pain.
- Fighting arthritis. [28]

And so much more! **We weren't meant to sit slumped at a desk or laid back on the couch all day.** *Our bodies were meant to move! Get up and get active!*

# Build Your Own Routine

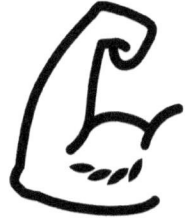

## Frequency

The first step to building your own training routine is determining the number of days per week that you'd like to work out. **Ideally, you should work out three to four times each week for 30-60 minutes each session.** The type of workouts you do will be based on your goals, lifestyle, and schedule.

If you don't have access to a gym, or you tend to travel a lot, then **calisthenics,**[22] resistance-band, and **HIIT**[23] workouts will be best. However, if you do have access to a gym and can go regularly, then gym-based weight training workouts with a blend of calisthenics and HIIT is the way to go. Of course, though, if you prefer at-home calisthenic workouts, then by all means do those at home.

## Split

Once you've decided on your workout frequency, next determine your workout split. Common program splits include:

### Three-Day
- Full-Body
- Lower/Upper/Full-Body

---

[22] *Body-weight exercises.*
[23] *High-Intensity Interval Training*

- Lower/Push/Pull

## Four-Day
- Full-Body
- Lower/Upper

## Five-Day
- Full-Body
- Lower/Upper + Full-Body
- Lower/Push/Pull/Lower/Upper

## Six-Day
- Lower/Push/Pull
- Chest/Back/Legs/Shoulders/Arms/Abs (aka, the *"Bro Split"*)

**The split you should choose is whatever works best for *you*.** If you're new a trainee, then a three-day full-body program is a great place to start. If you're more experienced and like working out more than three days each week, then go with a four-, five- or six-day routine. **But even if you've been training for years, if following a three-day split is more conducive to your lifestyle and schedule, then a three-day split is what you should follow.**

From my experience in both coaching clients and training for years myself; full-body, lower/upper, and lower/push/pull programs produce the best results in **hypertrophy**[24] and strength. The reason is that these splits allow you to train within the **ideal volume and frequency range of *40-70 reps per body part, two to three times per week.***

---

[24] *Muscle gain.*

Thus, although widely used by many, the *"Bro Split"* is actually the *least* effective because you're only training each body part once per week.

A typical training week on a **three-day program** will look like the following:

### Three-Day Full-Body Split

| Mon. | Tues. | Wed. | Thurs. | Fri. | Sat. | Sun. |
|------|-------|------|--------|------|------|------|
| Full | Off | Full | Off | Full | Off | Off |

For **four-day programs:** two days on, one day rest, two days on, two days rest works best.

### Four-Day Lower/Upper Split

| Mon. | Tues. | Wed. | Thurs. | Fri. | Sat. | Sun. |
|------|-------|------|--------|------|------|------|
| Lower | Upper | Off | Lower | Upper | Off | Off |

For **five-day programs:** you can go three days on, one day off, two days on, one day off; or all five days in a row with two consecutive days of rest is also good.

### Five-Day Lower/Push/Pull/Lower/Upper Split (1)

| Mon. | Tues. | Wed. | Thurs. | Fri. | Sat. | Sun. |
|------|-------|------|--------|------|------|------|
| Lower | Push | Pull | Off | Lower | Upper | Off |

### Five-Day Lower/Push/Pull/Lower/Upper Split (2)

| Mon. | Tues. | Wed. | Thurs. | Fri. | Sat. | Sun. |
|------|-------|------|--------|------|------|------|
| Lower | Push | Pull | Lower | Upper | Off | Off |

For **six-day programs:** you can go all six days in a row and rest the seventh—a typical lower/push/pull style; or you can go three days on, one day rest, repeat. Following this flow, however, would mean that you're actually only training six days per week every fourth week, and training five days each week for three weeks in a row.

## Six-Day Lower/Push/Pull Split

| Mon. | Tues. | Wed. | Thurs. | Fri. | Sat. | Sun. |
|------|-------|------|--------|------|------|------|
| Lower | Push | Pull | Lower | Push | Pull | Off |

## Five-Six Day Lower/Push/Pull/Rest Split

| Week | Mon. | Tues. | Wed. | Thurs. | Fri. | Sat. | Sun. |
|------|------|-------|------|--------|------|------|------|
| 1 | Lower | Push | Pull | Off | Lower | Pull | Pull |
| 2 | Off | Lower | Push | Pull | Off | Lower | Push |
| 3 | Pull | Off | Lower | Push | Pull | Off | Lower |
| 4 | Push | Pull | Off | Lower | Push | Pull | Off |

**Again, the split you choose comes down to whichever *you* prefer that best fits *your* schedule and level of training.**

## Reps & Sets

Depending on your goals, your reps per set and the number of total sets that you do per exercise will vary. Refer to the **Ideal Reps & Sets** table below.

## Ideal Reps & Sets

| Goal | Reps | Sets | Rest |
|------|------|------|------|
| Max Strength | 1-5 | 4-6 | 3-5 Minutes |
| Hypertrophy | 6-12 | 3-5 | 0-60 Seconds |
| Strength Endurance | 12-20 | 2-4 | 0-60 Seconds |

[25]

## Money Sets & Exertion

For how much you should lift per set, more often than not, you should work your way up until you're one to two reps shy of failure on your **money set.**

Your **money set** is *the set you do for each exercise where you attempt the most challenging weight or resistance to get stronger.* The sets leading up to your money set should be build-up sets with lighter but increasing weight, with a heavy focus on form.

For example, if you're doing three sets of 10 of a dumbbell bench press, then your money set would ideally be Set 3, with Sets 1 & 2 as build-ups. **The weight for your money set should be a weight that leaves you one to two reps shy of failure.** Meaning, for a set of 10, if you were to attempt an 11th or 12th rep, you'd fail and would have to drop the dumbbells or have your spotter help lift them up.

Thus, if the goal for your money set is the 60-pound dumbbells, then for your Set 1 build-up use the 50s, and for Set 2 the 55s. This slow increase in weight allows you to *"bridge-the-gap"* to your heaviest set, ensuring that your muscles (and mind) are thoroughly warmed and ready to lift the heavy load.

### Money Set Example

| Day 1 | | | | | | |
|---|---|---|---|---|---|---|
| Superset | Exercise | Reps | Set 1 | Set 2 | Set 3 | Rest |
| 1A | DB Bench Press | 10 | 50s | 55s | 60s | 0-60 sec. |

If you happen to fail on the 10th rep, that's okay because you're learning what your body is capable of. But don't go to failure on every set for every workout. **Going to failure is very taxing on the muscles, tendons,** joints, and nervous system. And doing so all the time will only hurt you in the long run, as your body won't ever fully recover.

So, although pushing to failure can be helpful at times when getting stronger; there's a time and a place for it (test days, burn-out and drop sets, etc.), and it shouldn't be a daily routine.

## Duration

**For the duration of your workouts, the common notion of *"more is better"* couldn't be further from the truth.** When resistance training, the body produces testosterone and human growth hormone (HGH). After 45 minutes of **anaerobic** exercise, it stops producing testosterone and HGH and instead starts producing cortisol. Testosterone and HGH are **anabolic**[25] **hormones,** meaning they **work** to *build* **muscle.** Cortisol, however, is **catabolic,**[26] meaning it *burns* **it.** [7]

And to be clear, **what I mean by exercise is *actual continuous exertion with minimal rest.*** I don't mean doing a set, and then checking Instagram for 10 minutes, doing a second set, and then talking to friends for another 10. If this is how you work out, then you won't need to worry about your body producing cortisol because it won't be stressed enough to produce any.

But assuming you *are* exercising with a purpose, **once you reach that 45-minute threshold, the stress of the workout will start to outpace the burning of carbs and fat for energy. As a result, the release of cortisol will cause the body to start burning muscle to meet its energy demands.** [7]

---

[25] *A state of growth within the body.*
[26] *A state of destruction within the body.*

Therefore, the ideal length of the resistance training portion for your workouts is 30-45 minutes. Any additional time for cardio, warm-up, and post-stretch is separate.

If you're max-strength training and doing low reps with heavy weight, your rest time between sets will be higher; meaning your workouts might extend to 45-60 minutes or longer. But other than that, 30-45 minutes is all you need.

### Ideal Workout Duration (Minutes)

| Warm-Up | Resistance Training | Post-Stretch | Cardio |
|---------|---------------------|--------------|--------|
| 5-10 | **30-45** | 5-10 | Discretionary |

## Variation

Because our bodies are designed to adapt and are very efficient at doing so, variance in your workouts is necessary for continuous progression, as the goal is **progressive overload:** *gradual increases in resistance used.*

This doesn't mean you have to completely switch up your routine, as you should always practice your main compound lifts each week (bench, deadlift, overhead press, pull-up, squat, etc.). But changes in the **acute variables** *(intensity, reps, sets, split, tempo;* especially the intensity), and your accessory exercises every two to four weeks will allow for this continued progression. [28]

For variation of intensity, some weeks you'll want to go:
- Low reps with heavy weight.
- Low reps with low weight.
- High reps with heavy weight.
- High reps with low weight.

The number of sets you do should also vary and, over time, so should the number of days per week that you train. This constant variation will force your body to continuously adapt, leading to continuous increases in muscle mass, strength, and fat loss. It'll also allow your body to properly recover during your weeks of less intense training, which will lead to further progression once you kick it up again.

## Effort

Not every workout will be your best, and not all need to be performed at a high intensity. But **to reach your full potential, *you should always be striving to get better*.** Whether with strength, conditioning, or simply form; your goal every workout should be to improve in at least one of these areas, if not all.

**Just going through the motions won't get the job done. If you want to build your dream physique, *then you have to put in the work*...Period!**

## Rest

**Equally significant to your time invested in the gym is your time spent on recovery.** When resistance training, you're breaking your muscles down and tearing muscle fibers. Through that break down of your muscles, you get bigger and grow stronger as your muscles repair themselves, which results in an increase in size and strength. However, without giving your body proper time to recover, this repair process will slow, or you'll simply plateau.

A great quote from my good friend and strength coach, Denzel Allen **(@powerofstrength),** is:

*"Hard work done 24/7 can't be hard work."*

If you're always working and never give yourself time to rest, you'll quickly burn out and only set yourself back. **This is precisely why** *working out every day is counter-intuitive, and you must take days off to recover.*

Personally, I prefer following a four-day lower/upper split. This allows me to train within the ideal volume and frequency range to see the results that I want while having plenty of time to recover with three days off each week to maximize performance.

It also allows me to include an optional fifth day, in which I'll do a full-body accessory workout focused on arms, core, calves, and conditioning, if I want; or have more time and energy for other activities like biking, hiking, snowboarding, and flag football–a few of my favorites.

## Cardio

As previously discussed, whether you prefer hitting the weights or doing calisthenics, **if you want a lean and muscular physique, then resistance training should always be your primary focus.** Unless, of course, your goal is to bike, run, swim, or anything of the sort for long distances, then long-distance conditioning is what you should do.

However, no matter your goal, building cardio into your routine helps for two reasons:
1. It improves your cardiovascular (heart) conditioning.
2. It increases your total calories burned.

There are two types of cardio:
1. **HIIT:** High-Intensity Interval Training
2. **LISS:** Low-Intensity Steady State

**HIIT** cardio is doing any exercise or series of exercises for a short duration of time (usually five- to 10-minute circuits or less) in a repeated work/rest interval fashion. Typically, intervals last for 10-60 seconds, and your work interval is generally the same length as your rest. During your work intervals, you're doing as many reps as possible (AMRAP) of your chosen exercise(s). Common HIIT exercises include:

- Battle ropes
- Jump rope
- Mountain climbers
- Sled push

But any other exercise that you'd like to do, whether calisthenics or using free weights, is also fair game.

**The target heart rate during HIIT work intervals is 70-90% of your max beats per minute (bpm), which is 220 minus your age. During your rest, it's 60-65%.** For example, at 25 years old, my max heart rate is 195 bpm; meaning my target work heart rate for HIIT workouts is 137-176 bpm, and my target rest heart rate is 117-127 bpm.

**Target Heart Rate Calculations**
- **Max Heart Rate:** 220 bpm - 25 years old = 195 bpm
- **Work Intervals**
  - 195 bpm × 0.7 = 137 bpm
  - 195 bpm × 0.9 = 176 bpm
- **Rest Intervals**
  - 195 bpm × 0.6 = 117 bpm
  - 195 bpm × 0.65 = 127 bpm

For example, at the end of your workout, you want to do three rounds of HIIT cardio with a work/rest interval of 30 seconds. Your exercise of choice is the battle ropes. Thus, for 30 seconds you'll do as many reps of battle ropes as possible; and then after 30 seconds has passed, you'll rest for another 30. After your 30 seconds of rest, you'll then repeat that cycle twice more to complete three rounds total.

### HIIT Workout Example

| Round | 1 | | 2 | | 3 | |
|---|---|---|---|---|---|---|
| Interval | Work | Rest | Work | Rest | Work | Rest |
| Time | 0:00-0:30 | 0:30-1:00 | 1:00-1:30 | 1:30-2:00 | 2:00-2:30 | 2:30-3:00 |

**LISS** cardio is doing any form of low-intensity movement at a steady pace for a long duration of time (usually 20-60 minutes or more). Typically, LISS cardio is done on machines like the:

- Elliptical
- Treadmill
- Stair Climber
- Stationary Bike

But biking, hiking, walking, and other low-intensity activities also count as LISS cardio, as well.

**The target heart rate for LISS cardio is 50-70% of your max bpm.**

Both types of cardio have their pros and cons.

**HIIT** cardio increases your metabolism after you've completed it (like resistance training), has a more profound effect on improving cardiovascular endurance and preserving muscle, and takes less time to do. However, it's more taxing on the body; and, if overdone, can delay recovery and lead to overtraining. This can result in injuries, increased muscle soreness, and progress plateaus. [28]

**LISS** cardio is less taxing on the body and increases your metabolism while doing it. However, it's more time-consuming; and, if overdone, can delay recovery, hinder muscle growth, and even decrease muscle mass. [28]

Which should you do, then? **Whichever *you* prefer that fits *your* goals.**

- Again, if your goal is to build a lean and muscular physique, then **HIIT** cardio is best.
- If you want to minimize your time spent doing cardio, then **HIIT** is also best.
- If you're dieting for fat loss and are in a consistent caloric deficit, then opt for more **LISS,** as it's less taxing on the body.
- **LISS** cardio should also be your go-to if your goal is long-distance training (biking, running, swimming, etc.).

But just like varying your training program helps with continued progression, the same applies to your cardio–*mix it up!* And, of course, *don't forget to include it!*

Whether you prefer doing a couple five- to 10-minute sessions of **HIIT** each week; 20- to 30-minute sessions of **LISS;** or becoming more active outside of the gym by doing other recreational activities; including cardio in your weekly routine will make you a healthier and better-conditioned person overall.

Plus, **cardio *in addition* to your resistance training allows you to eat more because it increases your total calories burned.**

For example, if your BWMC is 2,500, and your goal is one pound of fat loss per week, then your average daily calorie goal will be 2,000. However, if you do 25 minutes of LISS cardio after a workout and burn

250 calories while doing it, then you can eat an additional 250 calories and still maintain your 500-calorie deficit.

- **BWMC:** 2,500 kcals
- **1 lb. of fat loss per week**: BWMC - 500 kcals
- **2,500 kcals - 500 kcals** = 2,000 kcals
- **2,000 kcals - 250 kcals burned from LISS** = 1,750 kcals
- **1,750 kcals + 250 kcals extra food** = 2,000 kcals

The same thing applies if your goal is maintenance, but you want to eat more than your BWMC–**whatever additional cardio calories you burn can either be eaten to maintain your weight or deficit or used to create one if your goal is fat loss.**

Most importantly, though, **cardio improves your heart conditioning and your heart needs love, too. ;)**

## QUALITY Over Quantity

Above all, **the *most important* thing when exercising is your *form*.** Not only will poor form lead to less weight lifted; but it'll also lead to injury, which will only set you back from reaching your goals.

It doesn't matter how much the guy or girl next to you is lifting. If you can't lift the same weight with proper form and technique, *then don't try to!* This isn't a competition. The only person you're competing against is *yourself! **QUALITY** over quantity...always!*

At **Plant Strength Coaching,** we have a full exercise video library with 500+ exercises and variations showing you exactly how to perform each with proper form and technique. You'll receive access to all of this and more with your membership to our **Plant Strength Coaching App.** For more details, visit **plantstrength.com/coaching.**

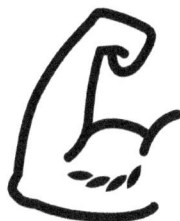

# Sample Program

Below is a sample three-day full-body program based on progressive overload. Week 1 has a strength endurance focus with higher reps, fewer sets, and lighter weight used; while Week 2 has a hypertrophy focus with fewer reps, more sets, and heavier weight used.

### Week 1: Strength Endurance

| Day 1 | | | | |
|---|---|---|---|---|
| **Superset** | **Exercise** | **Reps** | **Sets** | **Rest** |
| 1A | Back Squat | 12-15 | 2-3 | 0-60 sec. |
| 2A | Lat. Pull-Down | 12-15 | 2-3 | - |
| 2B | Hamstring Curls | 12-15 | 2-3 | - |
| 2C | Seated DB OH Press | 12-15 | 2-3 | 0-60 sec. |
| 3A | DB Bicep Curls | 12-15 | 2-3 | - |
| 3B | Cable Core Press (Each) | 6-8 | 2-3 | 0-60 sec. |

| Day 2 | | | | |
|---|---|---|---|---|
| 1A | Bench Press | 12-15 | 2-3 | 0-60 sec. |
| 2A | BB Hip Bridges | 12-15 | 2-3 | - |
| 2B | RC Face-Pulls | 12-15 | 2-3 | - |
| 2C | ALT DB Reverse Lunges (Each) | 8-12 | 2-3 | 0-60 sec. |
| 3A | RC Triceps Push-Downs | 12-15 | 2-3 | - |
| 3B | Reverse Crunches | 10-20 | 2-3 | 0-60 sec. |

| Day 3 | | | | |
|---|---|---|---|---|
| 1A | Deadlift | 12-15 | 2-3 | 0-60 sec. |
| 2A | Incline DB Bench Press | 12-15 | 2-3 | - |
| 2B | DB Step-Ups (Each) | 8-12 | 2-3 | - |
| 2C | SA DB Row (Each) | 8-12 | 2-3 | 0-60 sec. |
| 3A | DB Lateral Raises | 12-15 | 2-3 | - |
| 3B | Bicycles (Seconds) | 30-60 | 2-3 | 0-60 sec. |

## Week 2: Hypertrophy

| Day 1 | | | | |
|---|---|---|---|---|
| Superset | Exercise | Reps | Sets | Rest |
| 1A | Back Squat | 6-8 | 3-4 | 0-60 sec. |
| 2A | Lat. Pull-Down | 6-8 | 3-4 | - |
| 2B | Hamstring Curls | 6-8 | 3-4 | - |
| 2C | Seated DB OH Press | 6-8 | 3-4 | 0-60 sec. |
| 3A | DB Bicep Curls | 6-8 | 3-4 | - |
| 3B | Cable Core OH Press (Each) | 8-12 | 3-4 | 0-60 sec. |

| Day 2 | | | | |
|---|---|---|---|---|
| 1A | Bench Press | 6-8 | 3-4 | 0-60 sec. |
| 2A | BB Hip Bridges | 6-8 | 3-4 | - |
| 2B | RC Face-Pulls | 6-8 | 3-4 | - |
| 2C | Walking DB Lunges (Each) | 6-8 | 3-4 | 0-60 sec. |
| 3A | RC Triceps Push-Down | 6-8 | 3-4 | - |
| 3B | RC Crunches | 12-15 | 3-4 | 0-60 sec. |

| Day 3 | | | | |
|---|---|---|---|---|
| 1A | Deadlift | 6-8 | 3-4 | 0-60 sec. |
| 2A | Incline DB Bench Press | 6-8 | 3-4 | - |
| 2B | DB Side Step-Ups (Each) | 6-8 | 3-4 | - |
| 2C | SA DB Row (Each) | 6-8 | 3-4 | 0-60 sec. |
| 3A | DB Lateral Raises | 6-8 | 3-4 | - |
| 3B | Mountain Climbers (Seconds) | 30-60 | 3-4 | 0-60 sec. |

If you'd like to try out the **Plant Strength Coaching** platform, you can download this exact program by joining the **FREE Trial Group** via **plantstrength.com/coaching.**

In addition to the program above, by joining the free group, you'll also receive:

- Foam Roll, Dynamic Warm-Up & Post-Stretch Routines
- Full Video Exercise Library with 500+ Exercises & Variations
- Superset & Tempo Training Explanation Videos
- Plant Strength Coaching App (Available on the App Store & Google Play)
- 24/7 Support & FAQ Page

Part 8

# Putting It All Together

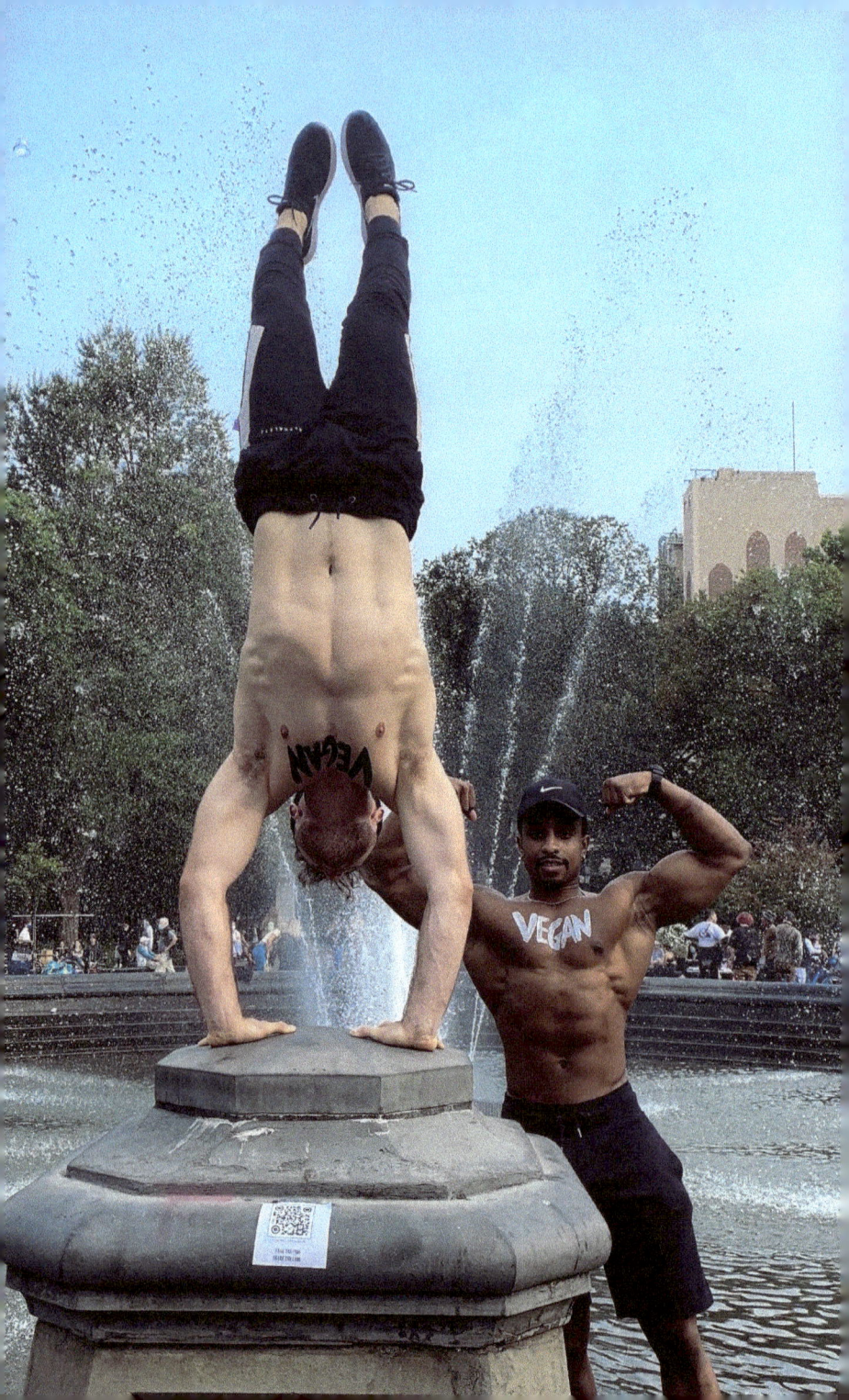

# Building Healthy Habits

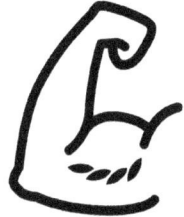

*"We are what we repeatedly do. Excellence then is not an act, but a habit."*

– Aristotle

Humans like comfort, which can make deviating from the norm difficult. However, **if you want to be successful in any aspect of your life, then you must take yourself out of your comfort zone, embrace new challenges, and build the healthy habits that produce *results that last!*** Below are the steps for how to do this.

## 1. Focus on *One* Habit at a Time

What many people do when they have many habits that they'd like to build or change, is they typically jump right in the deep end and try tackling everything at once.

- Exercise more often
- Reduce fast food intake
- Reduce soda consumption
- Sleep more
- Quit smoking

However, when this happens, these people usually start off well. But once the overwhelmed feeling sets in and the first setback happens, everything gets kicked to the curb and they fall right back into their old ways.

To avoid this, create a list of habits that you want to change and **begin with the *one* that you feel is most important.** Focus all of your efforts on that habit until you've mastered it and it becomes routine, then move on to the next.

## 2. Go Slow

Just like trying to change all of your habits at once, going from zero to 100 with even one of them can also be a recipe for failure.

If regular exercise is a habit that you'd like to build, but you haven't exercised regularly in months, then don't start by training four days each week for 60 minutes at a time. Instead, try starting with a 30-minute walk, two to three times each week. After that, slowly increase your activity from there.

If you'd like to decrease your fast food intake, but you currently frequent McDonald's, Burger King, and other similar restaurants three to four times each week, then start by cutting out one weekly visit. For example, instead of going four times this week, start by only going three. Then go only twice during next week, only once after that, once every other week; and so on and so forth. **Take small steps and eventually they'll turn into *giant* leaps!**

## 3. Write Everything Down

It's one thing to tell yourself what you're going to change and how you're going to change it, but it's another to **write down your goals and commit a plan to paper.**

If your goal is to reduce your soda consumption and, ultimately, cut soda out of your diet; then write down that goal and how you're going to do it, including:

- When you'll start and when you plan to be finished.
- How you'll track your progress.
- How you'll stay accountable.
- The people in your support system.
- What your motivators are.
- Possible obstacles to overcome.
- All of your triggers.

Put this plan in a place where you'll see it every day (on your fridge, next to your bed, etc.), then **stick to it!**

## 4. Create a Timetable

*"A goal without a deadline is just a dream."*

– Robert Herjavec

Once you choose your first habit to build, **set a date for when you'll start making changes and then another for when you want it built by.** Typically, 30 days is good a timeframe.

Doing so creates a deadline, which will help keep you focused and accountable. Think of it like project for work or school. When your boss or teacher says, *"Project A is due on the 30th,"* that means *Project A must be completely finished and submitted by the 30th* or else there'll be consequences (loss of job, bad grade, etc.). Holding yourself to a similar deadline when building a healthy habit will not only help you build it faster, but you'll also feel much more accomplished knowing that you were able to stick to your goal.

## 5. Track Your Progress

Although tracking your progress isn't necessary to build a habit, it helps keep you on task; just like creating a timetable for completion. **Maintaining a log of the progress you've made allows you to see how much you've actually done, and how far you still have to go.**

All of my clients use the **Plant Strength Coaching App** for their workouts to track the sets, reps, and weight used for every exercise of their program. I also have all of my clients submit progress pictures, track their food intake, and monitor their weight. We also keep a progress check-in log with personal notes from each coaching session to clearly see how far they've come.

## 6. Maintain Accountability

For some people, holding themselves accountable isn't a problem; but that's not the case for all. This is one of the main reasons why so many people hire coaches to help them reach their goals, as a good coach will hold them accountable. **Whether you hire a professional coach or seek the help of family members or friends, having someone to check in with makes a *huge* difference whenever you slack or lose motivation.**

Another great way to hold yourself accountable is to make your goals public. Just like writing your goals down makes them tangible, putting them out to the universe so that others can also see them *really makes them tangible!* Now, you'll have that many more people watching to see if you actually follow through. **In other words, *start posting to the gram! ;)***

## 7. Build Support

Support and accountability go hand-in-hand. Find that person or group of people (whether it's your best friend, sibling, a parent, people from an online forum all working towards a similar goal, etc.) who you can turn to when you need encouragement. Ask them to commit to helping you when needed and, in-return make the commitment to calling on them when times get tough.

## 8. Find Your Motivation

**With every goal, there's a reason for wanting to achieve it. And that reason is the driving force behind your motivation.** As we discussed in the "Mindset" section, when your motivation starts to wane (as it usually comes and goes), reminding yourself of the root reasons for why you're doing something will keep you committed to actually doing it.

**Dig deep and find your *"whys."* Your *"whys"* are what drive you.** Write them down and return to them as often as you need.

## 9. Think Through Obstacles

No path to success will ever be a straight line. **Any successful person will tell you that the journey to where they are today was filled with *many* setbacks and failures.** This is why thinking ahead about possible obstacles you may face along the way will make them easier to overcome when they arise.

If you're trying to reduce your alcohol consumption but tend to lose control when you go out with your friends, come up with a plan for what you'll do the next time you're out. For example, every time you buy a drink, you must also order a glass of water and finish that water before you can buy another. Hopefully, consuming the water will keep you full and discourage you from wanting to drink more.

If you have a sweet tooth (like me) and tend to get the sugar-cravings at night, try having a piece of fruit instead. This way, your sweet craving will be satisfied with a healthy option; and you'll no longer have the urge to raid the cookie jar.

## 10. Know Your Triggers

Every habit has its **habit triggers:** *events that immediately precede carrying out that habit.* Knowing your triggers will help break your bad habits, and you can then come up with positive ones for replacement.

As I just mentioned, I have the biggest sweet tooth. When it comes to baked goods and ice cream, you can always count on me to share some with you. With this sweet tooth, however, comes the tendency to overeat. Whenever I overconsume sweets, my triggers are usually that:

- I was starving and haven't eaten for a while.
- I was feeling *"some type of way"*–shout out Drake. ;)
- I was bored at home and not doing anything (which is usually never the case, as I always have something to do. But that's beside the point lol).

**To break my sweets-overeating habit, I've come up with positive habits to match all of my triggers.**

**If it's been a while since I've last eaten and my stomach is chomping at the bit, instead of going for the brownies on the counter, I eat some fruit or sweet vegetables (like carrots, peas, cherry tomatoes, etc.).** This way, I still get the sugar that my body's craving to raise my low blood sugar. The difference, though, is that it'll rise slowly (and not spike like it would with the brownies); as the sugar from the fruit and vegetables will gradually release into my bloodstream because of their slow-digesting fiber.

I'll typically combine the fruit and veggies with a protein shake, as well, which is filling and slow-digesting. However, if I'm still craving the brownies after the fruit, veggies, and shake; I'll go ahead and have one (or half of one). But the amount that I ultimately have will be far less than what I would have had if I hadn't had the nutrient-dense food beforehand.

**If I'm _"up in my feels"_ (which all of us are sometimes), I practice sitting with these feelings and meditating.** Without dwelling, I think about _why_ I'm feeling what I'm feeling and repeat to myself:

- _"This is only present-moment energy. These feelings will **not** last."_

This allows me to become more mindful of my emotions and understanding of my feelings instead of drowning them in pints of **Ben & Jerry's Non-Dairy Ice Cream (which, if I'm being completely honest, I still do sometimes lol).**

**If I'm bored at home and get the urge to raid the cabinets, fridge, and freezer; I leave my house and go for a walk.** I also make sure to bring a large water bottle with me and finish it before returning home, so I'll feel full when I get back. I'll likely take some fruit, veggies, or a protein shake with me, as well.

## 11. Stay Consistent

Once you know your triggers for the current habit that you're trying to change, and you've found replacement habits for when those triggers arise, **make sure to practice those replacement habits _every single time!_**

If you miss doing them once or twice, that's okay. Treat it as a setback and move forward. But if you regularly skip on your replacement habits, the more tempted you'll be to continue skipping them the next time your triggers arise. And the more you skip them, the further away you'll be from changing your bad habits, causing you to be stuck right where you started.

## 12. Stay Positive

**Never treat any setback as a failure. Instead, treat your** *"failures"* **as** *opportunities to learn.* When you skip a replacement habit, ask yourself:

- Why did I skip my replacement habit?
- What was I feeling at the time?
- Who was around me?
- Did I seek my support?
- What will I do differently next time around?

Evaluate every situation, **always look for ways to improve, and spin everything in a positive light.** Simply switching your thought process when having a setback from a negative stance such as, *"I'm a failure, I might as well give up,"* to a positive one like, *"I'm only human, let's see what I can learn from this experience to do better next time,"* will profoundly affect your level of success.

**We're all human.** *Nobody is perfect,* **and we** *all* **make mistakes.** But that's the beauty of it. **Mistakes make us** *better* **because they allow us to** *grow.*

**By changing your mindset, you'll** *CHANGE YOUR LIFE!*

## 13. Fully Commit

Write down the list of habits that you want to build or change, pick the *one* that's most important to you *now,* and go *all-in* on that habit and *that habit only.* Apply all twelve steps above, **trust the process, and** *never*

**give up! Stay *fully* committed, and only then will you achieve what you've always wanted!**

> *"Commitment and consistency: the difference between those who see results and those who stay the same."*

> – Bobby Lynch

Yes, I just quoted myself. ;)

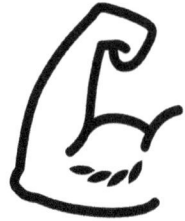

# Measuring Progress

## Progress Pictures

The first way to measure progress, which I feel is the *best* way, is through progress pictures. When you're making lasting changes to your physique, progress will be slow; and because you see yourself in the mirror every day, it'll be hard to notice the subtle differences.

On top of that, **the scale isn't always an accurate representation of the changes being made. If you lose five pounds of fat but gain five pounds of muscle, your weight will have stayed the same but the changes in your physique will be *enormous!***

Tracking your progress via pictures will give you a clear visual of the work you're putting in, allowing you to look back and see just how far you've come. **I recommend taking them every one to four weeks.**

## Measurable Statistics

The second way to measure progress is through measurable statistics, which include:
- Weight
- Body-Fat Percentage (BFP)
- Body-Circumference
- Performance

## Weight

Because the scale isn't always an accurate representation of progress, tracking your weight can help, especially if you're new to counting calories.

As previously discussed in the "Calorie Counting" chapter, to determine your Exact BWMC, you'll have to accurately count your calories for two weeks while tracking the daily changes in your weight. Unless you have elite-level goals (bodybuilding competition, weight-classed athletic event, etc.), **the number on the scale isn't that important.**

If your goal is to burn fat and build muscle to lead a healthier and happier life, then don't overly concern yourself with your weight. Weigh yourself once every one to two weeks to have an idea of where you're at; but remember, *your weight is just a number.* **Your BFP is what matters most.**

## Body-Fat Percentage (BFP)

Your weight comprises more than just fat. It also consists of muscle, bone, organs, water, food, glycogen, and more. And for most people, when they say they want to *"lose weight,"* what they're really saying is they want to *"lose fat."* Thus, tracking your BFP rather than only weighing yourself on the scale provides a much better measurable statistic of the changes in your physique.

**To track your BFP, you can use:**
- Visual Estimations
- Skin-Fold Calipers
- Bioelectrical Impedance (BIA)
- Bod Pod
- DEXA Scan

- Hydrostatic Weighing

The method you choose will depend on how much money you want to spend.

**Visual estimations** like you made when determining your protein-goal range (page 164) are free, and **skin-fold calipers** are cheap. So, if you don't want to spend a lot of money, then go with one of these. They do, however, provide the least-accurate results.

**Bioelectrical impedance analysis (BIA)** assesses your BFP by sending tiny electrical signals through your body and measuring how quickly they return. The more fat you have, the slower the current will be and the higher your BFP, and vice versa. Many at-home scales nowadays come with BIA technology to track your body composition, including your muscle mass, and cost anywhere from $50 to $100. Larger and more industrial BIA scales can also be found at many gyms and personal-training studios.

Although more accurate than the first two; your current hydration, fullness, and when you last exercised will affect the readings you get from BIA. This means you'll have varied results depending on when you test. When testing via BIA, it's best to do so in a fasted state while naked (or wearing only underwear) and first thing in the morning after using the bathroom.

**Bod Pod, DEXA Scan, and Hydrostatic Weighing** machines will produce the most accurate readings with a low percentage of error. And like BIA scales, they also measure your muscle mass, as well. However, these advanced measuring methods are only found in medical professional and lab-research settings, which makes them harder to access. They're also expensive and typically cost between $50 and $100 per test.

Healthy fat loss takes time. So, if you're measuring progress by tracking your BFP, test once every four to six weeks to see noticeable changes. And *always* **test using the same method for accurate comparisons.**

## Body Circumference

Measuring your body circumference in different areas is also a great way to track progress, if you're looking for measurable statistics. The most common areas to measure are your waist, hips, thighs, arms, and chest. Use a tape measure and have a coach, family member, or friend wrap it around each area and record your measurements. Again, as losing fat takes time, take these measurements only once every four to six weeks.

## Performance

Whether you're an athlete preparing for a sport or a person looking to get in better shape, **tracking your performance in the gym is the *best* way to measure progress statistically.** For every workout, record how much weight you lift and the number of reps you do for each set of every exercise. Each week that you revisit this exercise try to do *at least* the same amount of weight and corresponding reps as you did the previous week, or ideally a little more.

By tracking your workouts, you can see exactly how strong you're getting and also where you can still improve. The stronger you are, the more muscle you'll have relative to your body weight and the leaner you'll be even at a higher BFP. **More muscle also means a higher BWMC and faster metabolism.**

Constant improvement in strength and conditioning will ultimately translate into the results you want without the constant worry of whether or not your body numbers are changing. **Focus on getting better each and every day and let your results be the byproduct of the hard work you put in!**

All **Plant Strength Coaching** training programs are delivered through our **Plant Strength Coaching App** where you're able to track the sets, reps, and weight used for every exercise in your plan. To learn more, visit **plantstrength.com/coaching.**

**8.3**

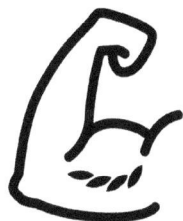

# Overcoming Plateaus

If your progress starts to slow or plateau, first off, ***DON'T STRESS!*** Stressing will *only make things worse.* Relax and understand that **plateaus are inevitable, and they happen to *everybody!***

Second, take a step back and assess the situation. Ask yourself:
- **How *much* am I eating–caloric intake?**
  - Calorie counting greatly helps with this (page 156).
- ***What* am I eating–80|20 Rule (page 154)?**
  - Am I eating enough lean protein and veggies?
  - Am I consuming enough fiber?
  - Am I drinking enough water?
  - Am I eating too many processed foods?
  - Am I drinking too many caloric drinks?
  - Am I cooking with too much oil or butter?
- ***How* am I eating–intuitively and mindfully (page 215)?**
  - Am I listening to my hunger and fullness cues?
  - Am I stopping when 70-80% full?
  - Am I consistently pushing past fullness?
- ***Why* am I eating–actually hungry, emotionally, socially?**
  - Am I eating because I'm *physically* hungry?
  - Am I eating out of boredom?
  - Am I eating to *"feel better"*?
  - Am I eating because other people are eating?
- **How much *effort* am I putting into my training (page 245)?**

- ○ Am I consistently pushing myself to get better every day?
- ○ Am I resistance training for at least 30-45 minutes, three times each week?
- ○ Am I doing any extra cardio or conditioning?
- ○ Am I living an active life overall (biking, hiking, swimming, recreational sports, etc.)?
- ○ Am I working out here and there, living mostly sedentary, and just going through the motions?
- **Am I doing all of the above consistently and well, 80% of the time?**

Remember, **what matters most for seeing changes in your physique is** *calories in versus calories burned.*

Therefore:
- **If your goal is to lose weight** but you're not losing any, then you're overeating.
- **If your goal is to gain weight** but you're not gaining any, then you're not eating enough.
- **If your goal is to maintain your weight** but you're either gaining or losing, then you're either overeating or undereating, respectively.

**How do you know whether you're eating too much or too little?** *By counting your calories.*

Although calorie counting isn't always necessary, and you can see results by solely intuitively eating, *it's an excellent learning tool.* Not only does it serve as a food diary that allows you to assess the nutrient density of your daily intake, but it also teaches you the calories and macros of the foods you regularly eat. And this is especially helpful if you've never counted before.

**If you're not currently counting, then I suggest doing so for a few weeks.** If your progress starts to pick up again, then continue counting if you wish or transition back to intuitively eating.

**However, if you *are* currently counting and your results keep stalling, then assess the accuracy of your counting.**
- Are you measuring or weighing all portions, including food, drinks, butter, oil, dressings, sauces, etc. (page 170)?
- Are you logging your food in its correct state–cooked vs. uncooked (page 195)?
- Are you crosschecking your macronutrients to ensure the app total is what your actual total is (page 176)?

**If you can answer *"no"* to one or more of these questions, then focus on improving here first.** Again, if after a few weeks you start seeing progress, then continue counting or transition back to intuitively eating. But if you don't see any progress, then you're still eating too much or too little.

**If this is the case, recalculate your BWMC using a new caloric multiplier (page 156).**
- Use a higher one if you're trying to gain.
- Use lower one if you're trying to lose.

Once you have your new BWMC, **add or subtract calories based on your goal.**
- Add calories to gain
- Subtract them to lose.

Continue making adjustments until your progress picks back up.

For *what* you're eating, keep your focus on nutrient-dense, plant-based foods (page 97); as these will provide your body with the vitamins, minerals, phytochemicals, and fiber that it needs for proper functioning and satiation. Again, I recommend calorie counting for a few weeks as a means of food journaling so that you can see what you're eating and if it's mostly healthy or not. Make adjustments as needed.

For *how* and *why* you're eating, calorie counting won't be helpful here. Refer back to the "Intuitive Eating" section (page 215), review how to eat intuitively, and then put the steps into practice.
1. Slow Down
2. Practice Noticing Your Cues
3. Use the Hunger & Fullness Scale
4. Journal
5. Meditate

For your training, focus on the base training tips outlined in the "Main Focus" chapter (page 280), or refer back to the "Training" section itself (page 233).

Just as eating well is essential, so is conditioning your body. Doing so will make everyday tasks a breeze; and you'll set yourself up for a healthy and long life. Moreover, **the more active you are and the more muscle you build, the faster your metabolism will be and the more you'll be able to eat; as muscle requires more calories to sustain itself than does fat.** *And who doesn't like to eat!?*

If you're currently not active enough, then start doing more. **You can expend more energy by:**
- Increasing the volume of each workout (the number of sets and exercises that you do).

- Pushing yourself harder by shortening rest times between sets and always trying to increase the amount of weight or resistance that you use *(with quality form)*.
- Including more cardio and conditioning in your routine.
- Becoming more active overall outside of the gym.
- Increasing **NEAT** *(Non-Exercise Activity Thermogenesis)* by, for example:
  o Using the stairs instead of the elevator.
  o Parking farther away from the store.
  o Getting a standing desk.
- All of the above.

Lastly and most importantly, **focus on doing all of the above consistently and well, 80% of the time.** Remember, **the goal *isn't* perfection; but what differentiates those who see results from those who stay the same is *commitment and consistency.***

In the short-term, the stock market notoriously goes up and down; but in the long-term, its trend is *always up.*

**Put your best effort forth and understand that you're human.**
- You'll make mistakes.
- You'll have setbacks.
- You'll have days of no motivation.
- And, at times, you may even feel like you want to quit.

But no matter what, ***NEVER GIVE UP! Forgive yourself, stay persistent, and be patient.* Your results *WILL* come. They'll just take time.**

# Transitioning to Veganism

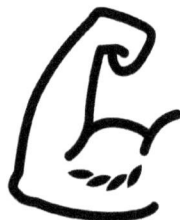

If you're looking to go vegan but are unsure what to do, simply start by swapping out the meat and animal products in your dish with a substitute. Many meat and animal product substitutes taste just as good as the real thing, *if not better!* Plus, *they're cruelty-free;* meaning no animal was harmed or killed in the making.

**My favorite meat- and animal-product-substitute brands are:**
- **Beyond Meat**
- **Boca**
- **Daiya**
- **Field Roast**
- **Follow Your Heart**
- **Gardein**
- **Lightlife**
- **Morningstar Farms**
- **Plant Strength** *(plantstrengthfoods.com)*
- **So Delicious**
- **Tofurky**

For example, start by taking your regular meat-potato-vegetable meal, like in the picture on the next page taken from my **Instagram (@bobbyphysique);** and, instead of eating meat, swap it out for a meat substitute. In this meal, I used **Morningstar Farms** chicken strips. For your potato, instead of loading it with butter, sour cream, and bacon bits, load it with black beans, salsa, and avocado, or eat it plain (like I do usually). Do the same for your veggies—eat them plain or zest them with lemon instead of butter.

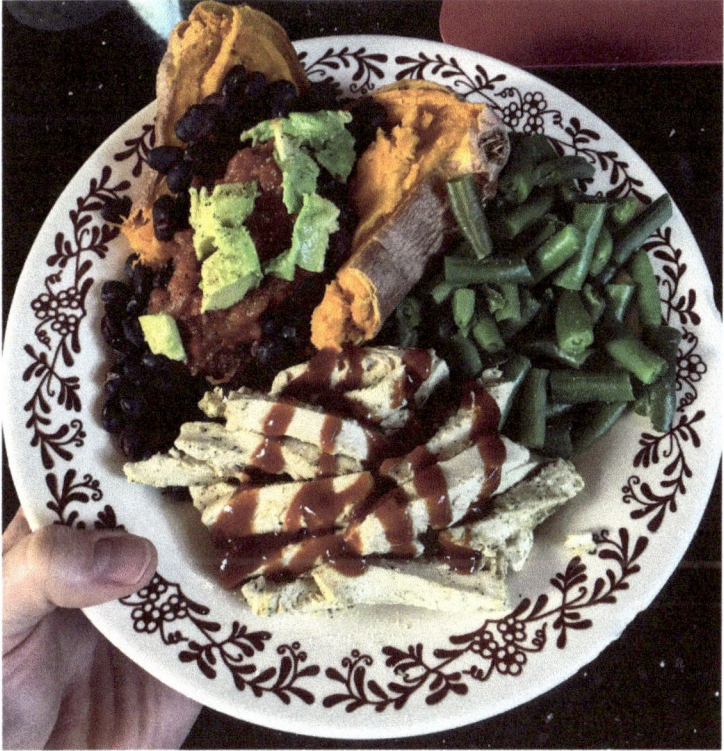

If you still really want to use butter or sour cream, then use a butter or sour cream substitute. **Earth Balance** makes a delicious vegan butter, plus many other vegan dressings and spreads.

After that:

- Focus on consuming more plant foods overall–fruit, veggies, leafy greens, whole grains, beans, legumes, nuts, seeds, etc. (See the "Best Nutrient-Dense Foods" list, page 97).
- Read ingredient labels and avoid foods containing meat, dairy, eggs, and any of the other non-vegan ingredients discussed in the "Grocery Shopping" chapter (page 117).
- Continue furthering your education on veganism and its positive effects (page 80).

*And that's it!*

**The beauty of today's day and age is that you can find a vegan alternative for practically *every* food, dish, liquid, snack, dessert; *you name it!***

Ideally, **your goal should be to consume as many natural foods as possible and minimize the number of processed ones that you consume; aka, *the 80|20 Rule* (page 154).** This *includes* processed mock-meat and animal-product alternatives, as some of them contain not-so-healthy additives and chemicals. But, for the sake of making the transition away from animal protein, substitutes are 100% the way to go!

I've become even *more* of a foodie since going vegan because it's forced me to get creative and try new things. I've also made so many of my own delicious meals, too, using my ***Buddha Bowl Blueprint*** (page 132).

And most importantly, when going vegan, always remind yourself of *why* you're making this transition; **whether it's for your health, the animals, the environment, or all three. Keeping your *"why"* in the forefront of your mind when tempted to eat meat or other animal products will make saying *"no"* that much easier.**

Continue doing this, and before you know it, you'll be fully vegan and *loving* the *amazing* benefits of a plant-based diet!

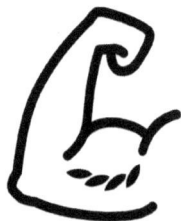

# Main Focus

Now that you've learned *everything* you need to know to not only see results but produce *results that last;* you're probably wondering what the next step is. We've covered so much in such a short amount of time that it probably feels overwhelming trying to process everything that you've just learned. But don't worry, *I GOT YOU!*

First and foremost, **start with your mindset (page 7).** Out of all the healthy habits that you can build, **a positive mindset is *by far* the healthiest!** Without one, even the smallest of tasks will seem daunting. Write out your goals, *"why's,"* and positive mantras; and repeat them to yourself every day. **Envision your success. Speak as if you're already where you want to be.**

Once you've opened your mind and have made it strong, create the list of habits that you'd like to build (page 257). Again, **start with the *one* that you feel is *most important.*** Focus on that habit and that habit alone and master it before moving on to another.

**If at any point you feel overwhelmed and want to quit, remember that it's *only* present-moment energy.** Take a step back, sit, meditate, recite your positive mantras, and remind yourself of *why* you're making a change.

For training and nutrition, focus on the base tips outlined below.

## Training

- **Have a plan.**
- *QUALITY* **over quantity.**
- **Lift heavy** (and under control).
- **Focus on compound lifts** (bench, deadlift, overhead press, pull-up, squat, etc.).
- Hours of cardio are *NOT* necessary to burn fat.
- **Resistance train** at least **three to four days each week** for **30-45 minutes per workout** (not including warm-up, post-stretch, or cardio).
- **Vary your routine** over time.
- **Get Better** *Every Day!*

## Nutrition

- **80|20 Rule:** 80% Nutrient-Dense Foods, 20% Empty Calories (page 154)
- **Eat intuitively** and listen to your hunger and fullness cues (page 215).
- **Count calories** as needed, especially if you've never counted before (page 156).
- **Workout Days:** More Protein and Carbs, Less Fat
- **Rest Days:** More Protein and Fat, Less Carbs (If Desired)
- **Drink LOTS of Water!**
  - **Men:** At least 1 gallon/day (128 oz.)
  - **Women:** At least 3/4th gallon/day (90 oz.)
- **Eat LOTS of Veggies!**
  - At least three (4 oz.) servings/day
- **When in doubt,** *lean protein and veggies.*
- **Batch Cook** (page 126) or **Meal Prep** (page 179) weekly.

- **Liquids:** Stick to only water, go with a diet or low-calorie option, or match each caloric drink with a glass of water (page 201).
- **Oil & Butter:** Avoid the use. At restaurants, ask for all meals to be prepared without oil or butter and to be steamed with water instead (page 201).
- **Dressings & Sauces:** Opt for the light option and minimize your portion size. At restaurants, ask for them on the side (page 202).
- **Fasting:** Fast for 12-16 hours following large calorically dense meals (page 203).

And last but not least, **stress less and *ENJOY LIFE!***

If you're not happy doing what you're doing, then chances of you continuing are slim. ***Don't restrict yourself.* Focus primarily on eating nutrient-dense, plant-based foods that'll make you feel, look, and perform your best. But also build in those empty calories you love!**

**Life is about *balance*.** The more balanced you are in all aspects of your life, the happier you'll be–*especially when it comes to food!*

Remember, this isn't a diet. ***It's a LIFESTYLE!***

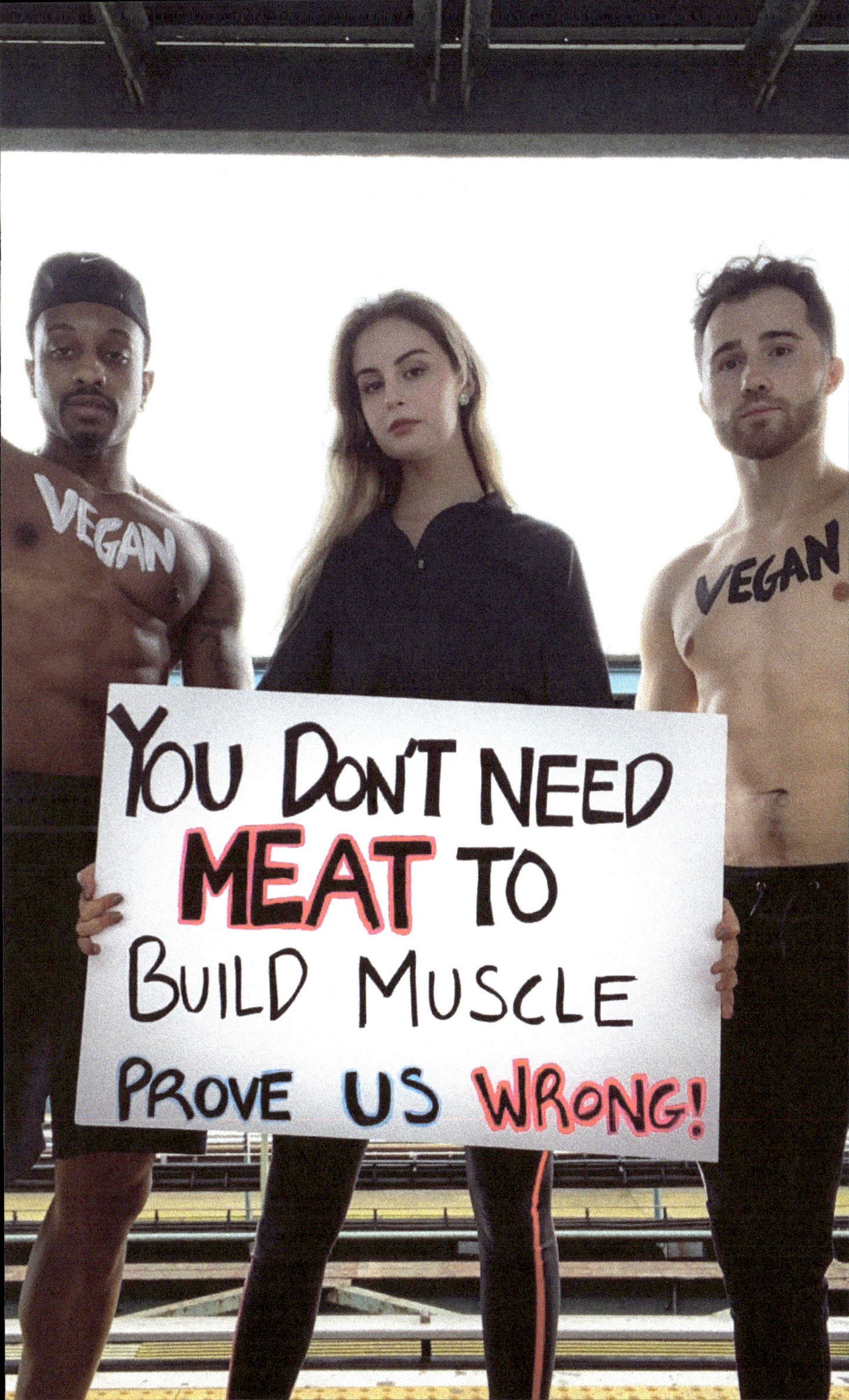

# Glossary

# XX

**80|20 Rule:** *At least 80% of your diet should be filled with nutrient-dense foods (see Nutrient Density) and the other 20% can come from empty calories (see Empty Calories).*

# A

**Aerobic Training:** *Conditions your slow-twitch (Type I) muscle fibers, which are large but thin. Examples include long-distance running, biking, walking, using an elliptical, etc. (see LISS).*
**Anabolic:** *A state of growth within the body.*
**Anaerobic Training:** *Conditions your fast-twitch (Type II) muscle fibers, which are smaller but dense. Examples include lifting weights, calisthenics, sprinting, HIIT cardio, etc. (see HIIT).*
**ATP:** *A molecule that moves energy to cells for muscle contraction (among other things).*

# B

**Basal Metabolic Rate (BMR):** *The amount of energy required to maintain vital bodily functions (breathing, pulse, blood flow, etc.) while in a resting state (sleeping or lying still).*
**Bioavailability:** *A measure of the absorption of nutrients by the body. The more bioavailable something is, the better the body absorbs it and vice versa.*
**Body-Weight Maintenance Calories (BWMC):** *The average daily number of calories required to maintain your current body weight.*
**Branched-Chain Amino Acids (BCAAs):** *Consist of the three essential amino acids leucine, isoleucine, and valine. Unlike the other six essential amino acids, BCAAs are mostly metabolized in the skeletal muscle rather than the liver. Because of this, their primary function is muscle protein synthesis (see Muscle Protein Synthesis).*

**Bycatch:** *The catch of non-target fish and ocean wildlife (seals, sea lions, dolphins, sharks, coral reef, etc.) including what is brought to port and discarded at sea.*

# C

**Cage-Free:** *See page 65.*
**Calisthenics:** *Body-weight exercises.*
**Catabolic:** *A state of destruction within the body.*

# D

**Diastolic Blood Pressure**: *The pressure in your blood vessels between beats.*

# E

**Empty Calories:** *Foods with low-nutritional value that are calorically dense; typically processed; and either very high in fat, preservatives, sodium, sugar, or all four.*

# F

**Flexible Dieting:** *Consuming a well-balanced, nutrient-dense diet without restrictions that consists of all the foods you love and enjoy.*
**Free-Range:** *See page 65.*

# G

**Grass-Fed:** *See page 65.*

# H

**Habit Triggers:** *Events that immediately precede carrying out that habit.*
**HIIT:** *High Intensity Interval Training*
**Homeostasis:** *A balance of energy in versus energy burned.*

**Hypertension:** *High blood pressure.*
**Hypertrophy:** *Muscle gain.*

# I

**Insulin:** *A storage hormone released by the pancreas when food is digested that's used to shuttle nutrients to your cells.*
**Intramyocellular Fat:** *The fat stored within the muscle tissue in your body that blocks the muscle's ability to uptake glucose, which then causes insulin resistance.*

# L

**Lean Body Weight (LBW):** *Your body weight minus your body fat (BW - BF).*
**LISS:** *Low-Intensity Steady State*

# M

**Money Set:** *The set you do for each exercise where you attempt the most challenging weight or resistance to get stronger.*
**Muscle Protein Synthesis:** *The process of building muscle, which not only builds it but also protects against its breakdown and damage.*

# N

**Non-Exercise Activity Thermogenesis (NEAT):** *The calories you burn during all activity other than purposeful exercise. For example, bouncing your leg while sitting in a chair, doing light chores around the house, walking upstairs, etc.*
**Nutrient Density:** *The nutrient content of a food, relative to its calories, based on the micronutrients (vitamins, minerals, and phytochemicals) that it provides to your body.*

**Nutrient Timing:** *The time during the day for when it's best to eat certain nutrients.*

## P

**Pasture-Raised:** *See page 65.*

**Phytochemicals:** *Biologically active compounds found only in plants, such as carotenoids, fiber, flavonoids, certain vitamins, and many other minerals that cannot be substituted through dietary supplements.*

**Progressive Overload:** *Gradual increases in resistance used.*

## S

**Systolic Blood Pressure:** *The pressure in your blood vessels when your heart beats.*

# References

[1]. A Calorie Counter. 2019. "USDA Nutrition Database." https://www.acaloriecounter.com.

[2]. Action Against Hunger. 2017. "World Hunger: Key Facts and Statistics." https://www.actionagainsthunger.org/world-hunger-facts-statistics?gclid=EAIaIQobChMI4K3j-uW-4AIVjZOzCh3k7QVHEAAYASAAEgIq8fD_BwE.

[3]. American Heart Association News. 2018. "More Than 100 Million Americans Have High Blood Pressure, AHA Says." January 31. *American Heart Association, Inc.* https://www.heart.org/en/news/2018/05/01/more-than-100-million-americans-have-high-blood-pressure-aha-says.

[4]. Andersen, Kip and Kuhn, Keegan. 2017. "Facts." *What The Health.* https://www.whatthehealthfilm.com/facts.

[5]. Andersen, Kip and Kuhn, Keegan. 2014. "The Facts." *Cowspiracy: The Sustainability Secret.* http://www.cowspiracy.com/facts.

[6]. Andrews, Ryan; Berardi, John; DePutter, Camille; Kollias, Helen; Scott-Dixon, Krista; and St. Pierre, Brian. 2017. "Forms." Toronto, Ontario. *Precision Nutrition, Inc.*

[7]. Andrews, Ryan; Berardi, John; DePutter, Camille; Kollias, Helen; Scott-Dixon, Krista; and St. Pierre, Brian. 2017. "The Essentials of Sport and Exercise Nutrition: Third Edition." Toronto, Ontario. *Precision Nutrition, Inc.*

[8]. Animal Clock. 2019. "2019 U.S. Animal Kill Clock." https://animalclock.org.

[9]. Animal Welfare Institute. 2018. "Inhumane Practices on Factory Farms." https://awionline.org/content/inhumane-practices-factory-farms.

[10].Bajpai, Prableen. 2019. "The World's Top 20 Economies." January 10. *Investopedia.* https://www.investopedia.com/insights/worlds-top-economies.

[11].Balentine, Jerry R. 2018. "Obesity." May 18. *MedicineNet.* https://www.medicinenet.com/obesity_weight_loss/article.htm#o besity_facts.

[12].Brogan, Gib; Cano-Stocco, Dominique; Enticknap, Ben; Hirshfield, Michael; Keledijan, Amanda; Lowell, Beth; Shester, Geoff; and Warrenchuk, Jon. 2014. "Wasted Catch: Unsolved Problems in U.S. Fisheries." March. *Oceana.* https://oceana.org/sites/default/files/reports/Bycatch_Report_FI NAL.pdf.

[13].Buettner, Dan. 2015. "The Blue Zones Solution: Eating and Living Like the World's Healthiest People." Washington, DC. *National Geographic Partners, LLC.*

[14].Buter, Terry; Fraser, Gary E.; Tonstad, Serena; and Yan, Ru. 2009. "Type of Vegetarian Diet, Body Weight, and Prevalence of Type 2 Diabetes." May. *Diabetes Care.* 32(5): 791-796. https://www.ncbi.nlm.nih.gov/pmc/articles/PMC2671114.

[15].Carlson, Richard. 1998. "Don't Worry, Make Money: Spiritual and Practical Ways to Create Abundance and More Fun in Your Life." New York, NY. *Hyperion.*

[16].Centers for Disease Control and Prevention. 2018. "Adult Obesity Facts." August 13. https://www.cdc.gov/obesity/data/adult.html.

[17].Centers for Disease Control and Prevention. 2017. "New CDC Report: More Than 100 Million Americans Have Diabetes or Prediabetes." July 18. https://www.cdc.gov/media/releases/2017/p0718-diabetes-report.html.

[18].Centers for Medicare & Medical Services. "NHE Fact Sheet." https://www.cms.gov/research-statistics-data-and-systems/statistics-trends-and-reports/nationalhealthexpenddata/nhe-fact-sheet.html.

[19]. Ciotti, Gregory. 2019. "The Most Important Mindset for Long-Term Success." *Sparring Mind.* https://www.sparringmind.com/growth-mindset.

[20]. Davis, Garth with Jacobson, Howard. 2015. "Proteinaholic: How Our Obsession with Meat Is Killing Us and What We Can Do About It." New York, NY. *HarperCollins.*

[21]. Dweck, Carol. 2010. "Change Your Mindset." *Mindset.* https://www.mindsetonline.com/changeyourmindset/natureofchange/index.html.

[22]. Dweck, Carol. 2010. "What is it?" *Mindset.* https://www.mindsetonline.com/whatisit/about/index.html.

[23]. Food & Water Watch. 2018. "Understand Food Labels." July 12. https://www.foodandwaterwatch.org/about/live-healthy/consumer-labels?gclid=EAIaIQobChMItafQpZW54AIVlIizCh2oeggTEAAYASAAEgK8lvD_BwE.

[24]. Hari, Vani. 2019. "Ingredients to Avoid in Processed Food." *Food Babe.* https://foodbabe.com/ingredients-to-avoid.

[25]. Hewlings, Susan J.; Horak, Adam; Kalman, Douglas S.; Klika, Brett; Lucett, Scott; McCall, Pete; Miller, Marty; Rhea, Matthew; Richey, Richard; Robles, Mabel J.; Stull, Kyle; Valency, Craig; and Weinberg, Robert. 2017. "NASM Essentials of Personal Fitness Training: Fifth Edition." Burlington, MA. *Jones & Bartlett Learning.*

[26]. Holt, S. H.; Miller, J. C.; and Petocz, P. 1997. "An Insulin Index of Foods: The Insulin Demand Generated by 1000-kJ portions of Common Foods." November 1. *The American Journal of Clinical Nutrition.* 66(5): 1264-1276. https://academic.oup.com/ajcn/article/66/5/1264/4655967.

[27]. Hyner, Christopher. 2015. "A Leading Cause of Everything: One Industry That Is Destroying Our Planet and Our Ability to Thrive

on It." October 23. *Georgetown Environmental Law Review.*
https://gelr.org/2015/10/23/a-leading-cause-of-everything-one-industry-that-is-destroying-our-planet-and-our-ability-to-thrive-on-it-georgetown-environmental-law-review.

[28].Joshi, Shivam. 2017. "Why Every Vegan and Vegetarian Needs Vitamin B12." August 31. *Forks Over Knives, LLC.*
https://www.forksoverknives.com/every-vegan-vegetarian-needs-vitamin-b12/#gs.0v5rbb.

[29].Kramer, Allyson. 2018. "7 Sneaky Non-Vegan Ingredients." December 27. *The Spruce Eats.*
https://www.thespruceeats.com/sneaky-non-vegan-ingredients-3371739.

[30].Lindsey, Rebecca. 2018. "Climate Change: Atmospheric Carbon Dioxide." August 1. *Climate.gov.* https://www.climate.gov/news-features/understanding-climate/climate-change-atmospheric-carbon-dioxide.

[31].Mickelson, Karen. "The Benefits of a Plant-Based Diet." *K's NRG Whole Food Energy Bars.* https://www.ks-nrg.com/why-vegan.

[32].Nordqvist, Christian. 2017. "How Useful is Body Mass (BMI)?" August 16. *Medical News Today.*
https://www.medicalnewstoday.com/articles/255712.php.

[33].Peta. 2019. "Factory Farming: Misery for Animals."
https://www.peta.org/issues/animals-used-for-food/factory-farming.

[34].Precision Nutrition. "Science or Fiction? Exploring the Benefits of Intermittent Fasting."
https://www.precisionnutrition.com/intermittent-fasting/benefits-of-fasting.

[35].Roach, John. 2006. "Seafood May Be Gone by 2048, Study Says." November 2. *National Geographic.*

https://www.nationalgeographic.com/animals/2006/11/seafood-biodiversity.

[36]. Sabet, Michael. 2010. "Understanding the Federal Commodity Checkoff Program." April. *Pennsylvania State University's Dickinson School of Law.*
https://pennstatelaw.psu.edu/_file/aglaw/Federal_Commodity_Checkoff_Program_Michael_Sabet.pdf.

[37]. Steele, Lauren. 2017. "This Guy Claims a Vegan Diet Cured His Colorectal Cancer-But Did It Really?" December 15. *Men's Health.* https://www.menshealth.com/health/a19545297/vegan-diet-cancer-cure.

[38]. The Vegan Society. 2019. "Vitamin D." *The Vegan Society.*
https://www.vegansociety.com/resources/nutrition-and-health/nutrients/vitamin-d.

[39]. Von Alt, Sarah. 2016. "WAKE UP! Tyson Dumps Over 6x More Toxic Pollution into Waterways Than Exxon." February 16. *Mercy For Animals.* https://mercyforanimals.org/wake-up-tyson-dumps-over-6x-more-toxic-pollution.

[40]. WW International, Inc. 2019. "Our Approach."
https://www.weightwatchers.com/us/our-approach.

# About the
# Author

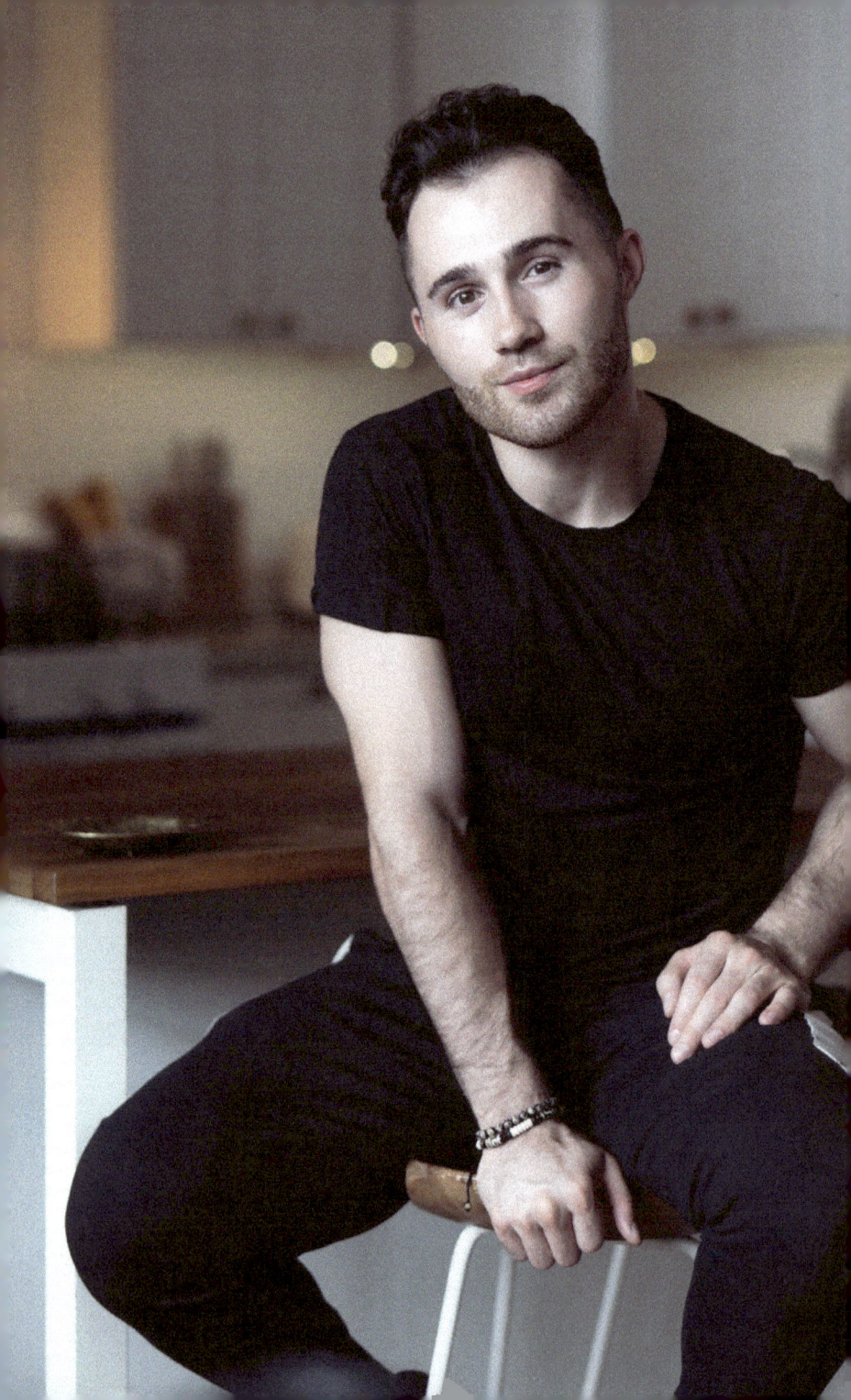

# Bobby Lynch

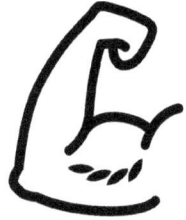

Bobby is a Certified Personal Trainer with the National Academy of Sports Medicine, a Professional Nutrition Coach with Precision Nutrition, and has a BA in Managerial Economics with a Minor in Spanish from Union College. As a vegan athlete and health coach, **his life mission is to *Defy The Status Quo* and show the world what's possible through *the power of plants!***

He is the Founder and CEO of the vegan company, **Plant Strength,** which supports *"sustainability for mind, body, soul, and the environment."*

He is the host of the podcast ***Plant Strength Radio*** and is an active public speaker who loves educating on the benefits of plant-based fitness and nutrition.

He's from Mystic, CT and finds much pleasure in traveling and immersing himself in the diverse cultures of the world.

**If you'd like to connect with Bobby,** you can find him on Facebook, Instagram, TikTok, Twitter, and YouTube **(@bobbyphysique),** where he provides free informative content to his followers.

**For business and speaking inquiries,** you may contact him directly by email at **bobby@plantstrength.com.**

**For coaching requests,** you may apply for a free consultation at **plantstrength.com/coaching.**

**plantstrength.com**

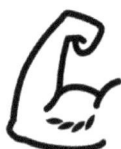

www.ingramcontent.com/pod-product-compliance
Lightning Source LLC
Chambersburg PA
CBHW041213030426
42336CB00023B/3327